THE QUICK & EASY
HEALTHY COOKBOOK

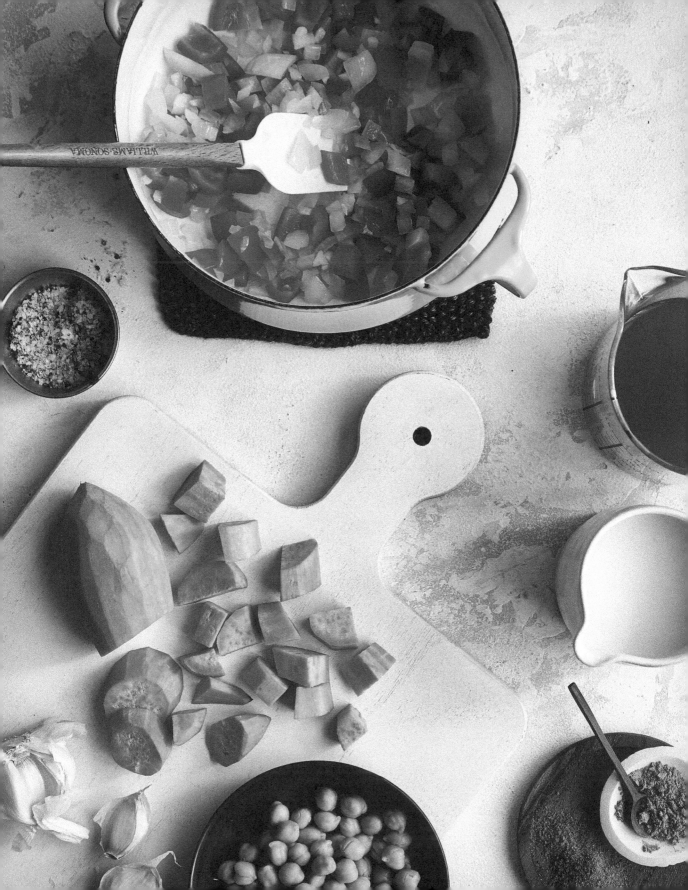

The Quick & Easy Healthy COOKBOOK

125 DELICIOUS RECIPES READY IN 30 MINUTES OR LESS

CARRIE FORREST, MBA, MPH

ROCKRIDGE
PRESS

For general information on our other products and services or to obtain technical support, please contact our Customer Care Department within the U.S. at (866) 744-2665, or outside the U.S. at (510) 253-0500.

Rockridge Press publishes its books in a variety of electronic and print formats. Some content that appears in print may not be available in electronic books, and vice versa.

Interior and Cover Designer: Mando Daniel
Art Producer: Janice Ackerman
Editor: Nora Spiegel
Production Editor: Matthew Burnett
Production Manager: Riley Hoffman

Photography: © 2019 Helene Dujardin. Food Styling by Anna Hampton

ISBN: Print 978-1-64152-963-1 | eBook 978-1-64152-964-8
R0

*This book is dedicated to the memory of my grandmother **Gwen Dixon**, whose kitchen was always warm, loving, and full of treats.*

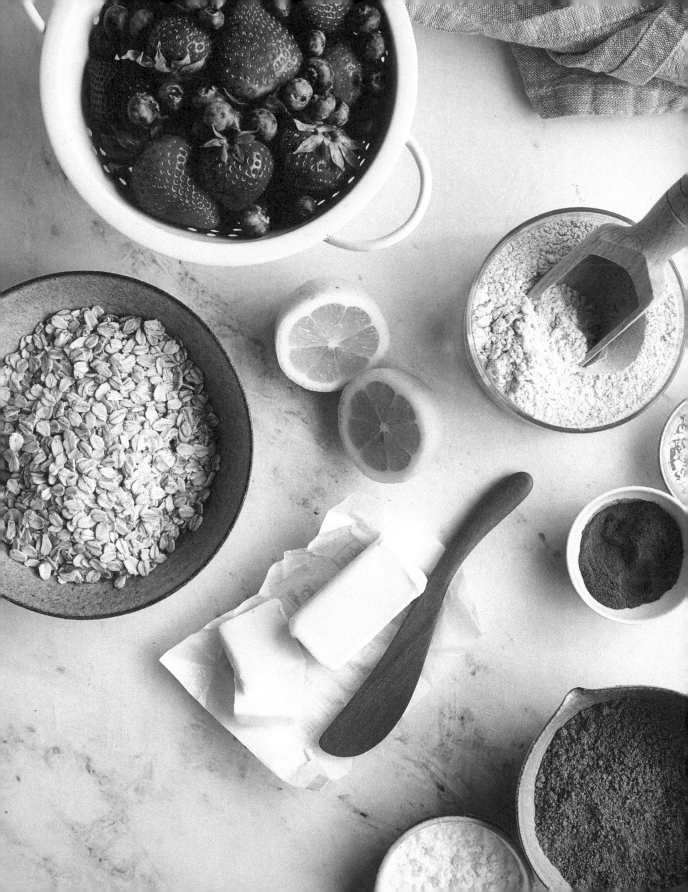

Contents

Introduction

There are so many reasons not to cook at home, from not knowing how or what to cook, to not having the right ingredients on hand, to simply not having time to spend in the kitchen. I understand how difficult it can be to get started, especially if you're used to grabbing fast or prepared foods.

I never learned how to cook in my younger years. I had a turbulent childhood with parents who were preoccupied with their own problems, including ongoing concerns about making ends meet. One of the ways in which I coped was by eating sugar and candy. I remember eating a lot of packaged foods, all the while failing to make any connection between what I ate and how I felt.

After I moved away from home, I got busy with school, and later with my career. I didn't learn to cook until my early thirties, instead relying on frozen or boxed meals. By that time I had developed a long list of health problems, including thyroid disease, autoimmune issues, polycystic ovary syndrome, digestive problems, migraines, chronic anxiety, allergies, and panic attacks. So, I learned the hard way that not spending the time preparing healthy meals can have devastating consequences. Then, in my midthirties, I was diagnosed with thyroid cancer. I felt as if my whole world was falling apart.

Following my cancer treatment and recovery, something shifted in the way I thought about food. It almost felt as if a light bulb had turned on in me. I started looking at food and ingredients as fuel for my recovery. Each meal became an opportunity to feel better. Over time, as I learned how to cook balanced meals and how to take better care of myself in general, my other troublesome symptoms diminished, and, in some cases, completely disappeared.

The good news is that you don't have to spend hours shopping, prepping, and cooking every day. With some basic planning, you can learn how to make healthy and delicious meals in 30 minutes or less. Granted, slowing down to prepare a meal can be challenging. On some days, it may feel easier to just slip through the drive-through for a quick bite on the go. But what I have learned after everything I have been through is that cooking is an act of love. When you take the time to prepare a meal for yourself, your family, or your friends, you're showing that you care about yourself and others. Cooking at home also allows you to save money and exercise control over the quality of ingredients.

Each of the 125 recipes in this book is required to both taste great and use whole food ingredients that are nourishing and promote good health. In addition, you'll find ingredients that are readily available at most grocery stores, without having to buy a bunch of obscure items that you may use only once. I've also included all the timesaving tricks I've learned over the years so you don't have to spend hours prepping and slaving over a hot stove.

I truly believe that there is no better time spent than in the kitchen preparing quick and easy healthy meals. There is no better time to begin than now. So, let's get started!

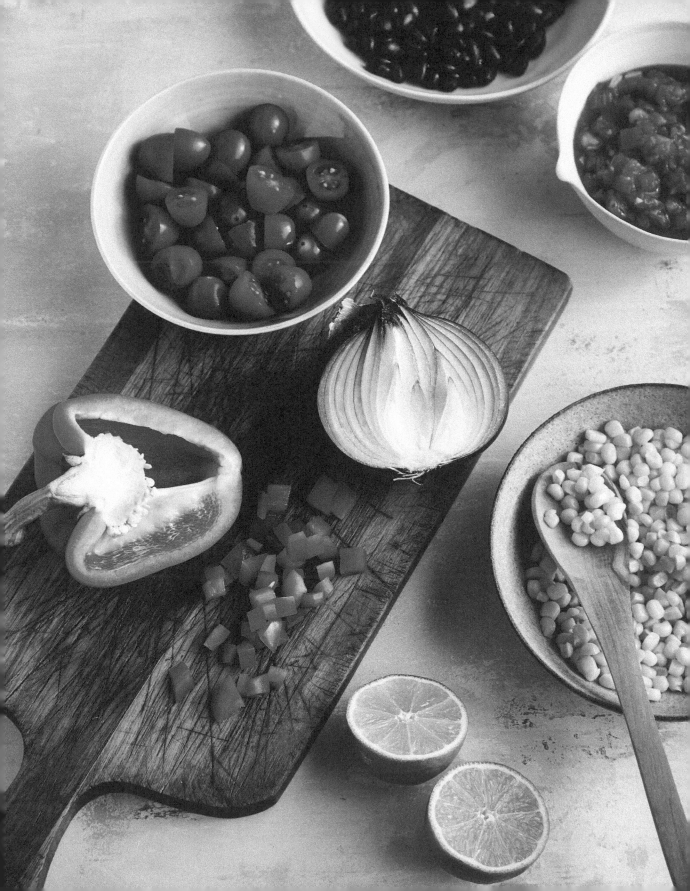

CHAPTER ONE

Quick & Easy Healthy Cooking

If you're new to healthy cooking, you might have confusion about what foods are considered healthy and how to use healthy ingredients to make dishes that taste good. Don't worry; you are in the right place. This chapter is a great starting point to learn about whole foods and how to incorporate them into your diet.

First we'll talk about what healthy cooking is and why it's important to cook with whole foods. It can be challenging to transition to a healthier diet, so I offer some tips to ease the transition. This chapter also includes meal-planning strategies, ideas to reduce food costs, tips for cooking efficiently, and ways to stock a healthy pantry.

Whether you're ready to make a big change or you're just looking to take baby steps into healthier eating, this chapter will give you all the tools you need to get started.

What Is Healthy Cooking?

Figuring out the healthiest ways to eat can be confusing. Everyone seems to have an opinion, and those opinions can sometimes be the opposite of one another. To keep it simple, I like to think of a healthy diet as one that includes as many whole foods as possible.

Whole foods are entirely natural, unprocessed ingredients. An example of a whole foods diet is one that includes proteins such as poultry, lean red meat, eggs, low-fat dairy, and fish; carbohydrates such as fruits, vegetables, whole grains, potatoes, and beans; and fats like butter, avocado oil, coconut oil, and olives or olive oil. Processing often strips otherwise healthy foods of their nutrition and adds a lot of unhealthy fat, salt, or sugar. For example, a baked potato is a whole food, but potato chips are a processed food. The goal for healthy cooking is to use ingredients that are in their whole food form.

What comes to mind when you think about healthy cooking? When I first began on my health journey, I thought that eating healthy foods meant eating boring, tasteless dishes that left me feeling unsatisfied and even hungrier than before. I can't count how many times I ate a plain green salad with fat-free dressing for dinner because I thought that was what eating healthy meant. The more I learned about nutrition, though, the more I realized that healthy cooking is more about incorporating a variety of real, whole foods into delicious, satisfying meals.

Now when I prepare meals, I make them balanced, with proteins, carbohydrates, and healthy fats. When I make salads, I've learned to top them with other healthy and nutritious foods, such as roasted sweet potato slices, shredded cooked chicken or turkey, chopped carrots, almonds, and sliced avocado. What once was a boring plate of greens is now a party of flavors and satisfying ingredients.

Using whole foods is actually a really fun, adventurous way of preparing healthy meals. The motto "eat the rainbow" is a great way of thinking about healthy cooking. Incorporating a variety of colors from fruits and vegetables ensures that you are getting lots of natural vitamins and minerals, which our bodies need to stay healthy. Fruits and vegetables in particular are a rich source of antioxidants, natural compounds that have been shown to fight cancer and help prevent disease.

One of my goals is to include at least one color of the rainbow, or at least one fruit or vegetable, into each meal. So, for example, a healthy breakfast could be a Strawberry-Banana Smoothie (page 16) or savory Cheesy Egg Muffins (page 18). The smoothie includes the color red from the strawberries, and the muffins include green and red from chopped spinach and red bell pepper. Thinking about how many colors of the rainbow you can eat in each meal is a fun challenge.

Here are some other ideas for how to get a variety of colors from whole foods into your diet:

Color	Food Examples
Red	Apples, beets, cherries, radishes, red bell peppers, raspberries, and tomatoes
Orange	Apricots, butternut squash, carrots, orange bell peppers, oranges, and sweet potatoes
Yellow	Corn, lemons, pineapple, spaghetti squash, and yellow bell peppers
Green	Avocado, asparagus, broccoli, celery, cucumbers, kiwi fruit, leafy greens such as spinach and kale, limes, peas, and zucchini
Blue & Purple	Blackberries, blueberries, eggplant, grapes, plums, prunes, and purple cabbage

Unless your doctor has prescribed you a certain diet, you don't have to think about healthy eating as being on a strict diet. A better way to think about healthy eating is to choose natural foods that will fuel your body for all of life's activities.

Why Whole Foods?

A whole foods diet includes more foods as found in their natural form and fewer processed foods from a package. By choosing whole foods as much as possible, you'll make it easier for your body to get the important nutrients it needs, including antioxidants and fiber. When you eat healthy foods, you'll also feel more satisfied after eating because your stomach isn't filling up just from a content standpoint, but also from a nutritional standpoint. What's more, eating a whole foods diet can save you money. When you plan your meals and prepare them at home, you are less likely to feel the urge to grab expensive prepared foods or sit down at a restaurant for a meal.

When visiting your grocery store, try sticking to the store's outer edges. This means shopping in the produce aisle or refrigerated meat and dairy sections for most of your foods. Try to stay away from the inner aisles, where the boxed, processed foods are typically found. However, frozen and canned whole foods can help stock a healthy pantry and keep your food costs down. While canned fruits and vegetables are processed and likely to include preservatives, this is minimal processing. And again, the goal of this diet is to eat more wholesome foods, not to strictly limit you in your grocery selection. Buying certain ingredients in bulk can also make budget sense. If you have a large freezer, having a big supply of staple fruits and vegetables can mean fewer trips to the grocery store as well.

Initially, the foods you make at home from whole ingredients may not taste as good as their processed versions because healthy recipes usually contain less salt and added sugars than processed foods. It can take a few weeks for your taste buds to adjust to a more wholesome diet, but rest assured that they will adjust.

Another challenge you might find is that you have to spend more time planning and shopping for groceries. If you are used to cooking out of a box or heating up a frozen meal, then it's important to schedule the time in your calendar to meal plan and shop. Even if initially it takes longer to shop for groceries, you'll find that over time your trips to the grocery store will be less time-consuming as your routine becomes more automatic and you learn to skip all the center aisles stocked with the processed foods.

Making It Quick & Easy

Numerous challenges can come up when you are trying to eat healthier. Some complaints about cooking I hear from my blog readers and friends are about the expense of cooking at home, the time it takes to cook, and a lack of cooking skills. These are all valid concerns. The good news is that with a little planning and effort and by using the skills outlined in this book, you will be on your way to making healthy meals fast, even if you're a beginner, have limited time, or are on a budget.

It's important to remember that the goal of a whole foods diet is not to make you feel guilty or restricted in your food choices, or leave you feeling hungry, but rather to gradually swap out processed foods for homemade meals made that will better fuel your body. You don't have to think about foods as being good or bad. Simply try to make choices that support how you want to feel, remembering that processed, prepared, and premade foods are generally higher in added sugars, fats, and sodium, and restaurants and manufacturers are concerned primarily with making food taste good, not preserving the healthy qualities of foods.

It does take more time to prepare and cook your meals than to buy them premade in a box or carton, but I think you'll find over time that it's generally less expensive, healthier, and not that difficult to cook your own meals at home. So try to plan to cook your own food whenever possible. Over time, you may even find that cooking is a good way to clear your mind after a long and busy day.

One way to find success in changing your diet is to take small steps toward a bigger goal: Start small. For example, if you normally skip breakfast and then grab something at a restaurant for lunch, try eating breakfast at home and taking your lunch to work twice a week. You could accomplish this goal by shopping on Sundays so you have the ingredients you need to make three recipes during the week. As you try out new recipes and find ones you like, you can increase the number of meals you prepare at home and reduce the number of meals you eat out.

This book will help you put healthy, great-tasting meals on the table in 30 minutes or less. I've used all the available shortcuts to reduce the time necessary to prepare and cook the recipes, without compromising on flavor or healthfulness. For example, I've reduced the time to bake chicken in the oven simply by cutting the chicken into cubes so it cooks in half the time. I think you'll find that once you've made some of the recipes in this book, you'll be able to take the skills you've learned and apply these time-saving techniques to your own dishes.

Tips to Make It Easier

Whether you're new to cooking or you're an expert in the kitchen, I hope you'll appreciate these tips, which are designed to make healthy cooking easy and efficient:

Make a weekly meal plan. Meal planning is one of the best things you can do to be successful with healthy eating. Use a whiteboard or a digital note-taking program to keep track of the meals you plan to serve each day.

Prepare ingredients ahead of time. You can buy ingredients prewashed and chopped, or set aside the time to organize and prepare your ingredients when you bring them home from the grocery store, so they are ready when it's time to cook. On busy days, knowing that you have everything you need ready to make a certain dish will make it much likelier that you'll follow through on cooking.

Shop smart. If you don't have time to waste in the grocery store, you can buy in bulk or order ingredients online. For the items you need to buy fresh at the store, make sure you have a list when you go, so you know exactly what you need.

Divide the work. Cooking with a partner or friend is a great way to ease the burden and make it more fun. You can get kids involved, too, by having them do age-appropriate tasks such as washing and peeling vegetables. It's also nice to have some help cleaning up.

Cook in bulk. Doubling a recipe and refrigerating or freezing the leftovers is a fantastic way to plan ahead. You can also bulk-cook staple items like rice and potatoes, and then serve them in different ways throughout the week.

Multitask with different appliances. Maximize your kitchen time by using different appliances at the same time to cook different foods. While you need only minimal appliances to make the recipes in this book, you can also branch out and try using a pressure cooker, slow cooker, or air fryer.

About the Recipes

This book contains 125 healthy recipes that can be made in less than 30 minutes from start to finish. The recipes call for using whole food ingredients you can find at most grocery stores.

To make the book easy to navigate, the recipes are organized into chapters by meal types and main ingredients. You'll find chapters dedicated to breakfast, soups and salads, snacks and sides, desserts, and basics and extras. For recipes based on specific ingredients or nutritional preferences, there are chapters for vegetarian mains, seafood, poultry, and meat.

Each recipe includes a yield and serving size, plus the active and total preparation time. I've also included labels to describe the dietary features of each recipe to make it easier for individuals with dietary restrictions:

- Nut-Free
- Gluten-Free
- Dairy-Free
- Soy-Free
- Vegetarian
- Vegan

To further help you find recipes that fit your needs, I've also tagged recipes with the following labels:

Extra Quick: These recipes can be made in 20 minutes or less. They are perfect for days when you are especially pressed for time and need a healthy meal extra fast.

Kids Love It: These recipes are more kid friendly. Examples include Blender Chocolate Chip–Oat Muffins (page 21), Healthy Baked Chicken Nuggets (page 80), and Spaghetti with Quick Bolognese (page 109).

Freezer Friendly: These recipes can be easily frozen and reheated at a later date. They make your life even easier by allowing you to store leftovers for future use.

The recipes in this book are casual, healthy, and full of flavor. I truly believe that there is something for everyone in this book. And they really do come together quickly. For example, here are three recipes that take fewer than 20 minutes each:

- Apple Pie Parfait (page 15)
- Sun-Dried Tomato and Hummus Quesadillas (page 44)
- Tuna-Stuffed Avocados (page 69)

There are plenty of vegetarian and vegan recipes in this book, too. For a plant-based day of eating, try the following:

- Vegan Tofu Scramble Breakfast Burritos (page 24)
- Lemon-Quinoa Vegetable Salad (page 33)
- Vegan Tempeh Tacos (page 53)

Lastly, if you're looking for healthy comfort foods, you might like these:

- Pumpkin Mac and Cheese (page 52)
- Barbecue Meatloaf Muffins (page 102)
- Edible Chocolate Chip Cookie Dough (page 134)

These are just a few examples of the variety of combinations you might make. Everyone has different preferences, so feel free to mix and match the recipes to develop a meal plan that works best for you. Start with recipes that use ingredients you love, because then you're more likely to actually follow through with making them. Pick one or two that sound good and create a shopping list to gather the ingredients you'll need to make those recipes.

Prepping Your Kitchen and Pantry

Being prepared is one of my best tips for healthy cooking. Make sure you always have the basics on hand to make your life easier when time is in short supply. I've pulled together some of my favorite kitchen tools and recommended ingredients so you can get started cooking as quickly as possible.

Top Five Kitchen Tools

You don't need a ton of special equipment to make the recipes in this book, but there are a few essential tools I recommend having:

Nonstick or Ceramic Cookware: At minimum, consider having a large skillet with a lid on hand. A large, lidded pot and a medium saucepan with a lid also are also useful. Several recipes in this book call for a muffin tin.

Baking Supplies: I recommend having at least one baking sheet that can withstand oven temperatures up to 450°F. Keeping parchment paper on hand for the baking sheet makes for an easy cleanup. Lastly, you'll need at least a couple of mixing bowls and at least one baking dish for many of the recipes in this book.

Wooden and Plastic Cutting Boards: A bamboo cutting board is useful for chopping vegetables. Add a couple of dishwasher-safe plastic cutting boards for prepping raw meat and poultry.

Chef and Paring Knives: You'll need, at minimum, a large chef's knife and a small paring knife.

Silicone and Stainless Steel Utensils: A serving spoon, spatula, ladle, colander, cheese grater, whisk, and tongs are essential utensils for your kitchen. I like to buy silicone or stainless steel utensils that can be washed in the dishwasher and handle heavy use.

Top Five Kitchen Appliances

Oven: Having a full-size oven with reliable temperature settings is important for cooking and is necessary to make a lot of the recipes in this book.

Stove Top: A gas or electric stove top with at least one burner is also required to make a majority of the recipes in this book.

Blender: While a blender is not required to make the majority of recipes in this book, having a modern, standard blender is nice if you want to make smoothies.

Food Processor: You don't need to invest in a food processor to make any of the recipes in this book, but they come in handy if you want to slice or grate vegetables quickly. You can also use a food processor to make sauces and salsas.

Juicer: I have both electric and manual juicers and use them often in my cooking. Fresh lemon or lime juice squeezed on top of most dishes adds flavor and brightness and helps reduce the amount of salt needed.

Recommended Pantry Items

It's a good idea to keep a stocked pantry so you have what you need to make healthy meals. I recommend having the following on hand to make most of the recipes in this book:

Baking Supplies: unsweetened applesauce, almond flour, cornstarch, chocolate chips, cocoa powder, whole wheat flour, vanilla extract, baking powder, and baking soda

Canned or Boxed Foods: tuna, beans, coconut milk, tomato paste and diced tomatoes, canned pumpkin, and low-sodium beef, chicken, or vegetable broths

Condiments: ketchup, reduced-sodium soy sauce, reduced-sodium tamari, hoisin sauce, mustard, apple cider vinegar, balsamic vinegar, and mayonnaise (look for mayonnaise brands made with coconut oil or avocado oil)

Cooking Oils: olive oil, coconut oil, nonstick cooking spray, and toasted sesame oil

Dried Herbs and Spices: black pepper, cayenne pepper, chili powder, ground cinnamon, ground cumin, curry powder, garlic powder, oregano, sea salt, thyme, and turmeric

Dried Fruits: raisins and dates

Grains: rolled oats, pastas, whole wheat bread crumbs, and quinoa

Nuts and Seeds: whole nuts and nut butters. (look for natural nut butters with no added sugars)

Sweeteners: coconut sugar, maple syrup, molasses, honey, and brown sugar

Now that we've covered the basics of healthy cooking and how it's possible to make delicious meals in 30 minutes or less, it's time to get started cooking.

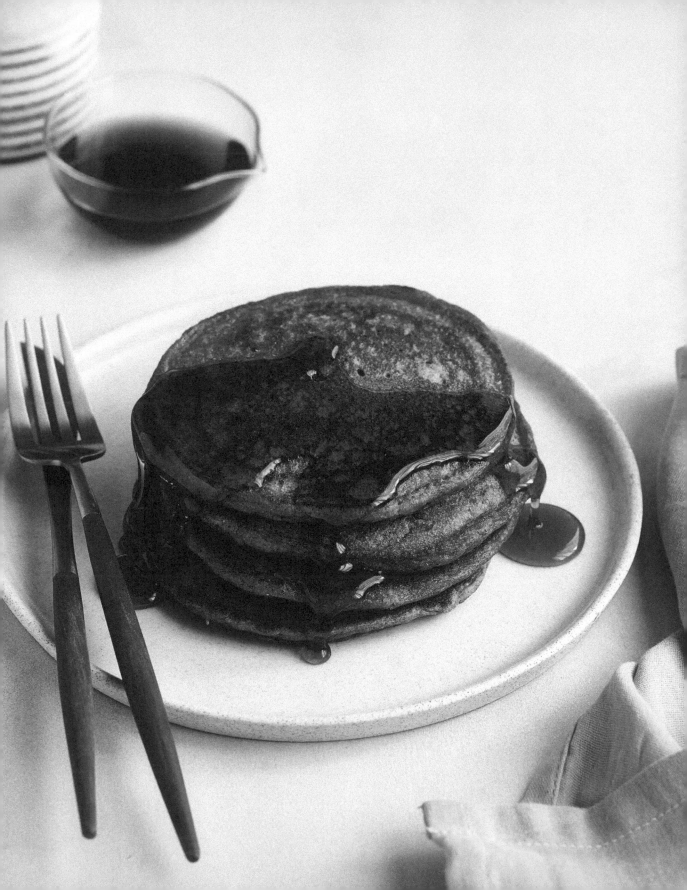

Breakfast

Whole Wheat Pumpkin Spice Pancakes

Loaded Sweet Potato Toasts

This recipe takes toast to the next level, using thin slices of sweet potato instead of bread. Trust me, you're going to love it. You can get creative with your toppings, choosing whatever fresh fruit is in season.

2 medium sweet potatoes

Nonstick cooking spray

4 tablespoons almond butter

1 banana, sliced

1 cup fresh strawberries, chopped

GLUTEN-FREE
DAIRY-FREE
SOY-FREE
VEGAN

Active Time: 15 minutes
Total Time: 30 minutes

Yield: 2 servings
Serving size: 4 slices

TIP: Choose medium sweet potatoes that are short and round, as opposed to long and thin. This will ensure that you get even-size toasts.

1. Preheat the oven to 400°F. Line a baking sheet with parchment paper and set it aside.

2. Scrub the sweet potatoes and pat them dry with a clean towel.

3. Cut the ends of each sweet potato, then use a sharp knife to carefully slice each potato lengthwise into long, round slices about ½ inch thick. You should get about four slices per sweet potato.

4. Lay each slice onto the baking sheet. Spray the tops lightly with nonstick cooking spray.

5. Place the baking sheet in the oven and bake for 20 minutes, or until the middle of the toasts have started to bubble, indicating that they are cooked through.

6. Remove the baking sheet and transfer the sweet potato toasts to a serving tray. Use a knife to spread ½ tablespoon of almond butter on each slice. Top with sliced banana and strawberries and serve immediately.

Per serving: Total calories: 406; total fat: 18g; saturated fat: 2g; carbohydrates: 58g; sugar: 18g; fiber: 11g; protein: 8g; sodium: 22mg; cholesterol: 0mg

Apple Pie Parfait

Yogurt parfaits are a great grab-and-go breakfast option. You can make them ahead of time if you know you're going to have a busy morning. This version is made using plain yogurt sweetened with maple syrup and is topped with crunchy apple and pecans. The protein in the yogurt makes this a satisfying breakfast with a flavor reminiscent of apple pie.

32 ounces plain, unsweetened yogurt (for vegan version, use dairy-free yogurt)

½ cup maple syrup

½ teaspoon ground cinnamon

½ teaspoon vanilla extract

1 apple, chopped

4 tablespoons almonds, chopped

GLUTEN-FREE
SOY-FREE
VEGAN
EXTRA QUICK
KIDS LOVE IT

Active Time: 15 minutes
Total Time: 15 minutes

1. Pour the yogurt into a medium mixing bowl. Stir in the maple syrup, cinnamon, and vanilla.

2. Use a serving spoon to divide the yogurt between four containers and top with the chopped apple and almonds.

3. Serve immediately, or cover and refrigerate for up to 4 days.

Yield: 4 servings
Serving size: 1¼ cups

TIP: Make these parfaits in small jars with lids for easy portability as a grab-and-go meal or snack.

Per serving: Total calories: 293; total fat: 3g; saturated fat: <1g; carbohydrates: 52g; sugar: 45g; fiber: 2g; protein: 14g; sodium: 204mg; cholesterol: 5mg

Strawberry-Banana Smoothie

I make a smoothie for breakfast most days of the week, and this recipe is one of my favorites. The color of this smoothie will be green from the spinach, but I promise you won't feel as if you're drinking raw spinach. It tastes like a tart strawberry milkshake, and it's rich, creamy, and so satisfying.

1 cup milk (for vegan option, use plain, unsweetened almond milk)

1 cup plain yogurt (for vegan option, use dairy-free yogurt)

2 tablespoons maple syrup

2 cups baby spinach

1½ cups frozen strawberries

1 banana

NUT-FREE
GLUTEN-FREE
SOY-FREE
VEGAN
EXTRA QUICK

Active Time: 10 minutes
Total Time: 10 minutes

Yield: **2 servings**
Serving size: **1½ cups**

TIP: For extra richness and flavor, add 2 tablespoons of peanut butter to the mixture before blending.

1. Put the milk, yogurt, maple syrup, and spinach into the pitcher of your blender. Blend the ingredients on high for 30 seconds.

2. Add the strawberries and banana to the pitcher and blend them on high for 1 minute more. If necessary, stop the blender and use a spatula to push the fruit down toward the blade to ensure that the ingredients get completely blended together.

3. Divide the smoothie between two glasses and serve immediately.

Per serving: Total calories: 281; total fat: 4g; saturated fat: 2g; carbohydrates: 53g; sugar: 39g; fiber: 5g; protein: 13g; sodium: 186mg; cholesterol: 15mg

Chocolate-Cherry Smoothie

If you've ever had a Black Forest cake, you know that chocolate and cherries make a killer combination. This smoothie is a healthy way to enjoy that flavor for breakfast. Frozen cherries and cocoa powder blended together make this smoothie a decadent treat.

---

1 cup milk (for vegan option, use unsweetened almond milk)

1 cup plain yogurt (for vegan option, use dairy-free yogurt)

2 cups frozen sweet cherries

2 pitted Medjool dates

3 tablespoons cocoa powder

¼ cup almond butter

GLUTEN-FREE
SOY-FREE
VEGAN
EXTRA QUICK
KIDS LOVE IT

Active Time: 10 minutes
Total Time: 10 minutes

---

1. Combine the milk, yogurt, frozen cherries, dates, cocoa powder, and almond butter in the pitcher of your blender. Blend the ingredients on high for 1 minute.

2. Divide the mixture between two glasses and serve immediately.

Yield: 2 servings
Serving size: 1½ cups

TIP: If you want to prepare this recipe ahead of time, combine all the ingredients except for the frozen cherries in your blender pitcher and store in the refrigerator. Then, when you're ready to make it, add the frozen cherries and blend.

Per serving: Total calories: 427; total fat: 22g; saturated fat: 4g; carbohydrates: 47g; sugar: 34g; fiber: 9g; protein: 19g; sodium: 151mg; cholesterol: 15mg

Cheesy Egg Muffins

If you like the flavor of quiche, you'll really like these egg muffins. They're crustless and get baked right in a muffin tin. The combination of egg, veggies, and melted cheese is such a tasty and satisfying way to start the day.

Nonstick cooking spray

9 eggs, lightly beaten

1 red bell pepper, chopped

1 cup baby spinach, chopped

½ cup shredded Cheddar cheese

¼ teaspoon sea salt

¼ teaspoon freshly ground black pepper

NUT-FREE
GLUTEN-FREE
SOY-FREE
VEGETARIAN

Active Time: 10 minutes
Total Time: 30 minutes

Yield: 4 servings
Serving size: 3 muffins

TIP: These muffins can be reheated in the microwave. Put them on a microwave-safe plate and heat for 20 to 30 seconds, or until hot.

1. Preheat the oven to 350°F. Lightly spray a 12-cup muffin tin with nonstick cooking spray and set aside.

2. Combine the eggs, bell pepper, spinach, cheese, salt, and black pepper in a large mixing bowl. Stir the ingredients gently to combine.

3. Fill each muffin cup carefully about three-quarters full, leaving room for the muffins to rise.

4. Bake the muffins for 20 minutes, or until the centers of the muffins have set. Let cool slightly before removing from the pan.

5. Serve immediately.

Per serving: Total calories: 228; total fat: 15g; saturated fat: 7g; carbohydrates: 4g; sugar: 1g; fiber: 1g; protein: 18g; sodium: 405mg; cholesterol: 431mg

Peanut Butter Oatmeal

One of my favorite snacks growing up was peanut butter and honey on a piece of toast. This homemade oatmeal recipe is reminiscent of that childhood favorite but transformed into a satisfying breakfast. The banana, raisins, and honey all add to the sweetness of this creamy, rich oatmeal.

1¾ cup milk (for vegan option, use plain, unsweetened almond milk)

2 cups gluten-free rolled oats

1 banana, sliced

¼ cup natural peanut butter

2 tablespoons honey (for vegan option, use maple syrup)

2 tablespoons raisins

½ teaspoon ground cinnamon

GLUTEN-FREE
SOY-FREE
VEGAN
EXTRA QUICK
KIDS LOVE IT

Active Time: 10 minutes
Total Time: 20 minutes

Yield: 4 servings
Serving size: 1 cup

1. Pour in the milk into a medium saucepan. Turn the heat to medium-high and bring the milk to a simmer.

2. Turn the heat to low and stir in the rolled oats and banana. Stir consistently for 1 minute so the banana starts to dissolve into the oats and milk.

3. Cover the pot and cook for 8 minutes on low heat.

4. Stir in the peanut butter, honey, raisins, and cinnamon and serve immediately.

Per serving: Total calories: 371; total fat: 12g; saturated fat: 2g; carbohydrates: 54g; sugar: 21g; fiber: 6g; protein: 13g; sodium: 114mg; cholesterol: 7mg

Breakfast Bacon-Sausage Patties

These homemade bacon-sausage patties are ridiculously good. They're made with ground pork and chopped bacon and are easy to throw together and cook on the stove top. You can serve them with scrambled eggs, toast, and hash browns, or entirely on their own.

1 pound ground pork

4 slices uncooked bacon, chopped

1 teaspoon onion powder

½ teaspoon garlic powder

½ teaspoon dried thyme

½ teaspoon ground cinnamon

¼ teaspoon freshly ground black pepper

NUT-FREE
GLUTEN-FREE
DAIRY-FREE
SOY-FREE
FREEZER FRIENDLY

Active Time: 15 minutes
Total Time: 25 minutes

Yield: 4 servings
Serving size: 2 patties

1. Line a plate with paper towels and set aside.
2. In a large bowl, combine the pork, bacon, onion powder, garlic powder, thyme, cinnamon, and pepper.
3. Use your hands to mix the ingredients together and form 8 patties. Flatten the patties so they cook evenly.
4. Heat a large nonstick skillet over medium heat. Put the patties in the skillet and cook for 4 minutes on each side.
5. Once they are fully cooked, use a spatula to transfer them to the plate to absorb any excess grease. Serve hot.

TIP: You can freeze any leftover cooked sausage patties in an airtight container or zip-top bag for up to 2 months. Reheat them in the microwave or on the stove top.

Per serving: Total calories: 346; total fat: 27g; saturated fat: 10g; carbohydrates: 1g; sugar: <1g; fiber: <1g; protein: 23g; sodium: 226mg; cholesterol: 92mg

Blender Chocolate Chip–Oat Muffins

What could be easier than making muffins in a blender? This recipe is designed to get the muffins in the oven as quickly as possible. Then, once they're done baking, you can pop them out of the muffin tin and eat them while the chocolate chips are melty and delicious. These muffins are not too sweet and have lots of fiber, making them a perfect breakfast dish.

Nonstick cooking spray

2 bananas

2 eggs

2¼ cups gluten-free rolled oats

⅓ cup plain unsweetened almond milk

⅓ cup honey

⅓ cup natural peanut butter

1 teaspoon vanilla extract

1 teaspoon baking powder

½ cup dairy-free chocolate chips

GLUTEN-FREE
DAIRY-FREE
SOY-FREE
VEGETARIAN
KIDS LOVE IT
FREEZER FRIENDLY

Active Time: 10 minutes
Total Time: 30 minutes

Yield: 12 muffins
Serving size: 2 muffins

TIP: To freeze any leftovers, let the muffins cool completely. Put them in a zip-top bag and freeze for up to 2 months. Defrost the muffins in the refrigerator and reheat them in the microwave for 20 to 30 seconds before serving.

1. Preheat the oven to 375°F. Spray a 12-cup muffin tin with nonstick cooking spray and set aside.

2. Combine the bananas, eggs, oats, almond milk, honey, peanut butter, vanilla, and baking powder in the pitcher of your blender. Blend on high to a smooth consistency.

3. Add the chocolate chips into the blender and use a spatula to stir them in.

4. Pour the batter into the muffin tin, leaving a little bit of room in each cup for the muffins to rise.

5. Bake for 20 minutes, or until a toothpick inserted in the center comes out clean. Let the muffins cool for a few minutes before removing from the tray.

6. Store any leftover muffins in the refrigerator for up to 5 days.

Per serving: Total calories: 216; total fat: 9g; saturated fat: 3g; carbohydrates: 30g; sugar: 15g; fiber: 3g; protein: 6g; sodium: 44mg; cholesterol: 31mg

Baked Denver Frittata

Eggs are such a great breakfast food, and this oven-baked frittata is an easy and hands-off way to make them. With precooked ham, cheese, and lots of vegetables, this is a hearty dish that will keep you satisfied for hours. It's easy enough to make on a weekday, but fancy enough to serve for Sunday brunch.

1 tablespoon olive oil

1 red bell
pepper, chopped

1 green bell
pepper, chopped

½ onion, chopped

8 eggs

⅓ cup milk

1 cup shredded
Cheddar cheese

1 cup chopped
cooked ham (omit for
vegan option)

Salsa for topping
(optional)

NUT-FREE
GLUTEN-FREE
SOY-FREE
VEGAN

Active Time: 10 minutes
Total Time: 30 minutes

Yield: 4 servings
Serving size: 1 piece

1. Preheat the oven to 400°F.

2. Heat the olive oil in a 10-inch oven-safe skillet over medium heat.

3. Put the bell peppers and onion in the skillet, sautéing for 3 minutes.

4. In a large mixing bowl, whisk together the eggs and milk.

5. Add the cheese and ham to the egg mixture and stir to combine.

6. Pour the egg mixture into the skillet and stir gently to combine with the sautéed peppers and onions.

7. Transfer the skillet to the oven and bake for 20 minutes, or until the center of the frittata has set.

8. Remove the skillet from the oven when the frittata has finished cooking.

9. Slice the frittata and serve hot with a dollop of salsa on top, if desired.

Per serving: Total calories: 375; total fat: 26g; saturated fat: 11g; carbohydrates: 8g; sugar: 3g; fiber: 1g; protein: 26g; sodium: 778mg; cholesterol: 418mg

Whole Wheat Pumpkin Spice Pancakes

Almost everyone loves pancakes for breakfast, and this recipe is sure to be a favorite. The canned pumpkin replaces the fat found in typical pancake recipes and also adds nutrition and a cozy fall flavor. The whole wheat flour makes them even more wholesome, with a subtle nutty taste.

1¼ cups milk

1 cup canned pumpkin

1 egg

1 teaspoon vanilla extract

2 tablespoons unsalted butter, melted

1 cup whole wheat flour

2 teaspoons baking powder

2 teaspoons ground cinnamon

Nonstick cooking spray

1 cup maple syrup, for topping

NUT-FREE
SOY-FREE
VEGETARIAN
KIDS LOVE IT
FREEZER FRIENDLY

Active Time: 20 minutes

Total Time: 30 minutes

Yield: 2 servings
Serving size: 4 pancakes

1. In a large mixing bowl, combine the milk, canned pumpkin, egg, vanilla, and melted butter. Use a whisk to gently combine.

2. Add the flour, baking powder, and cinnamon. Use a spatula to combine.

3. Heat a griddle over medium heat, and coat it lightly with nonstick cooking spray.

4. Use a ¼-cup measure to pour the batter onto the griddle, leaving plenty of room between each pancake.

5. Cook for 3 minutes, or until small bubbles start to appear in the batter. Flip each pancake over. Cook for an additional 3 minutes. Use a spatula to move the cooked pancakes to a plate.

6. Serve hot, topped with maple syrup.

TIPS: This recipe can be easily doubled or tripled to yield more servings. If you need to work in batches, set your oven to 200°F or its lowest setting. Keep the cooked pancakes on an oven-safe plate in the oven to keep them warm until you've finished cooking.

If you have any leftovers, you can freeze them in a zip-top bag for up to 2 months. Defrost them in the refrigerator for at least 12 hours prior to serving. Reheat the defrosted pancakes in a toaster oven.

Per serving without maple syrup: Total calories: 460; total fat: 17g; saturated fat: 9g; carbohydrates: 65g; sugar: 11g; fiber: 14g; protein: 18g; sodium: 203mg; cholesterol: 133mg

Vegan Tofu Scramble Breakfast Burrito

These vegan breakfast burritos have tons of flavor and nutrition. The tofu adds a healthy serving of plant-based protein, and the sautéed vegetables, avocado, and salsa give them a Mexican flair. You can make the burritos to order, or prepare them ahead of time, wrap them in foil, and warm them in the oven just before serving.

1 tablespoon olive oil

1 onion, chopped

1 red bell pepper, chopped

½ teaspoon sea salt

1 pound extra firm tofu, drained and chopped

1 teaspoon ground cumin

1 teaspoon ground turmeric

4 flour tortillas, warmed

1 avocado, pitted, peeled, and sliced

½ cup salsa

NUT-FREE
GLUTEN-FREE
DAIRY-FREE
VEGAN

Active Time: 30 minutes
Total Time: 30 minutes

Yield: 4 servings
Serving size: 1 burrito

TIP: It's best to use extra firm tofu for this recipe so it is not too watery. Unlike other types of tofu, extra firm tofu does not need to be pressed before using.

1. In a medium skillet, heat the olive oil over medium heat.

2. Add the onion, red bell pepper, and salt.

3. Use a spatula to stir the ingredients. Cook the vegetables for about 5 minutes, or until the onion starts to soften.

4. Add the tofu, cumin, and turmeric, stirring to combine. Cook for 5 minutes more so the tofu warms all the way through.

5. Put the warm tortillas on a flat surface when you're ready to serve the dish. Add a scoop of the scramble mixture to each tortilla, along with a few slices of avocado and a scoop of salsa.

6. Fold each burrito into a wrap and cover with foil to keep warm for serving.

Per serving: Total calories: 344; total fat: 18g; saturated fat: 3g; carbohydrates: 32g; sugar: 3g; fiber: 7g; protein: 17g; sodium: 609mg; cholesterol: 0mg

Cinnamon-Raisin Breakfast Cookies

What could be tastier than cookies for breakfast? These breakfast cookies are lightly sweetened with honey and raisins, rich in fiber, and full of cinnamon flavor. Keep them in the refrigerator and grab a couple on your way out the door. They also make an excellent healthy snack.

1¼ cups whole wheat flour

1 cup rolled oats

1 cup raisins

1 teaspoon ground cinnamon

1 teaspoon baking powder

¼ teaspoon sea salt

1 egg, lightly beaten

1 teaspoon vanilla extract

½ cup unsweetened applesauce

½ cup honey

¼ cup coconut oil, melted

NUT-FREE
DAIRY-FREE
SOY-FREE
VEGETARIAN
KIDS LOVE IT
FREEZER FRIENDLY

Active Time: 10 minutes

Total Time: 30 minutes

Yield: 12 cookies
Serving size: 2 cookies

TIP: These cookies freeze really well. Wait until they are completely cool before putting in a zip-top bag. You can store them for up to 2 months.

1. Preheat the oven to 350°F. Line two baking sheets with parchment paper and set aside.

2. In a large mixing bowl, whisk together the flour, oats, raisins, cinnamon, baking powder, and salt.

3. Add the egg, vanilla, applesauce, honey, and coconut oil to the bowl and stir to combine.

4. Scoop out tablespoons of dough and place them onto the baking sheets. You should fit about 6 cookies per sheet.

5. Bake the cookies for 20 minutes, or until the tops of the cookies have started to brown on all sides. Let cool slightly before serving.

Per serving: Total calories: 198; total fat: 6g; saturated fat: 4g; carbohydrates: 36g; sugar: 20g; fiber: 3g; protein: 4g; sodium: 57mg; cholesterol: 16mg

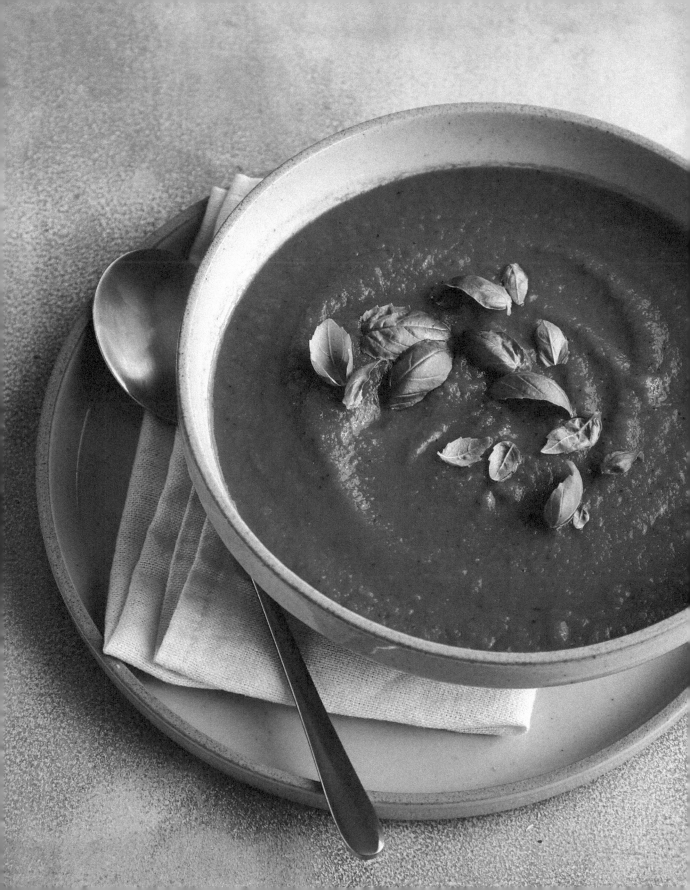

CHAPTER THREE

Soups & Salads

Creamy Vegan Blender Tomato Soup

Creamy Vegan Blender Tomato Soup

I published an almost identical version of this recipe on my website, Clean Eating Kitchen, and my readers went crazy over it. Nobody could believe how creamy this dairy-free, vegan soup turned out. The secret is using avocado instead of heavy cream. The soup is rich with tomato flavor and is one of my favorite easy lunch recipes.

2 (14.5-ounce) cans stewed tomatoes, with juices

1 avocado, pitted, peeled and halved

½ cup filtered water

½ teaspoon dried thyme

½ teaspoon dried basil

NUT-FREE
GLUTEN-FREE
DAIRY-FREE
SOY-FREE
VEGAN
EXTRA QUICK

Active Time: 5 minutes
Total Time: 10 minutes

Yield: 4 servings
Serving size: 1 cup

1. Combine the tomatoes, avocado, water, thyme, and basil in the pitcher of your blender. Blend on high until the mixture is smooth.

2. Pour the mixture into a medium saucepan over medium heat. Put a lid on the saucepan in case the soup starts to splatter. Let the soup come to a simmer.

3. Serve hot.

Per serving: Total calories: 131; total fat: 7g; saturated fat: 1g; carbohydrates: 18g; sugar: 8g; fiber: 5g; protein: 3g; sodium: 497mg; cholesterol: 0mg

Balsamic Beet Salad on Arugula

This salad includes a few shortcuts to make it really fast to make, including using preroasted beets and prewashed arugula. Beets are naturally sweet and become even sweeter when they are roasted. The beets balance the pepperiness of the arugula and the goat cheese adds nice creaminess. This is a great salad to serve at a dinner party.

1 (10-ounce) bag prewashed arugula

1 (8.8-ounce) package roasted beets, drained and sliced

3 ounces goat cheese, crumbled

¼ cup walnuts, chopped

¼ cup olive oil

2 tablespoons balsamic vinegar

1 teaspoon Dijon mustard

½ teaspoon freshly ground black pepper

GLUTEN-FREE
SOY-FREE
VEGETARIAN
EXTRA QUICK

Active Time: 15 minutes
Total Time: 15 minutes

Yield: 4 servings
Serving size: 1 cup

TIP: Look in the refrigerated section of your grocery store for packaged, roasted beets.

1. Put the arugula in a large mixing bowl. Add the beets, goat cheese, and walnuts and toss to combine.

2. In a small mixing bowl, combine the olive oil, balsamic vinegar, mustard, and black pepper. Whisk to combine.

3. Pour the dressing over the salad and give it a toss using tongs. Serve immediately.

Per serving: Total calories: 275; total fat: 24g; saturated fat: 6g; carbohydrates: 10g; sugar: 6g; fiber: 4g; protein: 8g; sodium: 214mg; cholesterol: 27mg

Curry Chicken Salad

Everyone who tries this dish loves it because it's both creamy and sweet, with the wonderful flavor of curry. You can serve it on toasted bread in a sandwich or by itself. I especially love the crunchiness of the celery, along with the texture from the raisins and grapes.

3 cups cooked chicken breast, chopped into bite-size pieces (for vegan option, use 1 pound extra firm tofu chopped into bite-size pieces)

3 celery stalks, chopped

¼ cup raisins

1 cup green grapes, halved

½ cup mayonnaise (for vegan option, use vegan mayonnaise)

Juice of 1 lemon

2 teaspoons curry powder

¼ teaspoon sea salt

¼ teaspoon ground black pepper

NUT-FREE
GLUTEN-FREE
DAIRY-FREE
SOY-FREE
VEGAN
EXTRA QUICK

Active Time: 10 minutes
Total Time: 10 minutes

Yield: 4 servings
Serving size: 1 cup

1. In a large mixing bowl, combine the chicken, celery, raisins, grapes, mayonnaise, lemon juice, curry powder, salt, and pepper. Stir to combine.

2. Serve at room temperature or chilled.

Per serving: Total calories: 443; total fat: 28g; saturated fat: 5g; carbohydrates: 19g; sugar: 15g; fiber: 3g; protein: 30g; sodium: 395mg; cholesterol: 86mg

TIP: You can substitute dried cranberries for the raisins to add a more tart flavor to the salad. Also, to save time, you can pre-cook the chicken to use on this salad. Herbed Cubed Chicken (page 153) is a good recipe to use for this.

Waldorf Chicken Salad with Chopped Apples, Grapes, and Walnuts

This salad was originally created at the turn of the nineteenth century by the maître d' at the Waldorf Astoria hotel in New York City. My husband and I visited the hotel a few years ago and loved the old-fashioned interior of both the hotel and restaurant. The salad has tons of flavor and texture, with a creamy dressing made from mayonnaise. I like to serve it on delicate butter lettuce.

3 cups chicken, diced and cooked (for vegan option, use 1 pound extra firm tofu, chopped)

1 cup green grapes, halved

3 celery stalks, chopped

1 apple, chopped

⅓ cup walnuts, chopped

⅓ cup mayonnaise (for vegan option, use vegan mayonnaise)

Juice of 1 lemon

1 head butter lettuce, leaves separated

GLUTEN-FREE
GLUTEN-FREE
DAIRY-FREE
SOY-FREE
VEGAN
EXTRA QUICK

Active Time: 20 minutes
Total Time: 20 minutes

Yield: 4 servings
Serving size: 1 cup

TIP: For the precooked chicken, try the Herbed Cubed Chicken (page 153).

1. In a medium mixing bowl, combine the chicken, grapes, celery, apple, and walnuts. Stir to combine.

2. In a small mixing bowl, mix the mayonnaise and lemon juice, using a spoon to stir the ingredients together.

3. Pour the dressing over the chicken mixture and stir to combine.

4. Put a few leaves of lettuce on each plate when you're ready to serve this dish. Spoon about 1 cup of salad onto the lettuce. You can serve the salad at room temperature or chilled.

Per serving: Total calories: 445; total fat: 28g; saturated fat: 5g; carbohydrates: 20g; sugar: 14g; fiber: 5g; protein: 32g; sodium: 204mg; cholesterol: 84mg

Italian Pasta Salad

A staple in Italian delis, this classic salad is flavorful and one of my go-to favorites. You'll get salami and olives in each bite, along with healthy chopped vegetables. This salad is great for when you need to pack a lunch that can be eaten at room temperature or chilled.

12 ounces uncooked rotini pasta (for gluten-free option, use gluten-free pasta)

1 cucumber, peeled and chopped

1 orange or yellow bell pepper, chopped

1 (6-ounce) can sliced black olives, drained

1 (4-ounce) package salami, chopped

Juice of 1 lemon

2 tablespoons olive oil

2 teaspoons dried Italian seasoning

NUT-FREE
GLUTEN-FREE
DAIRY-FREE
SOY-FREE
KIDS LOVE IT

Active Time: 15 minutes
Total Time: 25 minutes

Yield: 4 servings
Serving size: 1 cup

1. Bring 8 cups of water to a boil in a large pot. Add the pasta, lower the heat, and cover the pot.

2. Cook the pasta for 10 minutes over low heat. When the pasta is done cooking, drain in a large colander.

3. In a large mixing bowl, combine the cooked pasta, cucumber, bell pepper, olives, salami, lemon juice, olive oil, and Italian seasoning. Toss to combine.

4. Serve warm or chilled.

TIP: If you don't have Italian seasoning, you can substitute ½ teaspoon dried oregano, ½ teaspoon dried thyme, ½ teaspoon dried rosemary, and ½ teaspoon dried basil.

Per serving: Total calories: 544; total fat: 23g; saturated fat: 5g; carbohydrates: 75g; sugar: 2g; fiber: 4g; protein: 13g; sodium: 745mg; cholesterol: 22mg

Lemon-Quinoa Vegetable Salad

This bright recipe makes the perfect lunch to take to work or eat on the road. In fact, it's one of the recipes that I make the most often when I'm traveling. I like to make it the day before and pack it in a lightweight bowl with a lid. I find that this salad is flavorful and hearty but not too heavy. The fresh lemon adds brightness and helps bring all the ingredients together.

1 cup uncooked quinoa

2 cups reduced-sodium vegetable broth

¼ cup pine nuts

1 red bell pepper, chopped

1 cucumber, peeled and chopped

2 tablespoons olive oil

Juice of 1 lemon

¼ teaspoon fine sea salt

⅛ teaspoon freshly ground black pepper

GLUTEN-FREE
DAIRY-FREE
SOY-FREE
VEGAN

Active Time: 15 minutes
Total Time: 30 minutes

Yield: 4 servings
Serving size: 1 cup

1. Rinse the quinoa in a fine-mesh sieve until the water runs clear. Drain and put the quinoa in a medium saucepan. Add the broth and bring to a boil. Turn the heat to low, cover the pot, and let cook for 20 minutes.

2. While the quinoa cooks, toast the pine nuts in a small, dry skillet over low heat for 3 minutes. Once the nuts are done toasting, turn off the heat and set the skillet aside.

3. Turn off the heat under the quinoa once it's finished cooking, when the quinoa has absorbed all the water. Remove the lid and use a fork to fluff the cooked quinoa.

4. Transfer the cooked quinoa to a large mixing bowl. Add the red bell pepper, cucumber, pine nuts, olive oil, lemon juice, salt, and pepper. Stir to combine.

5. Serve chilled or at room temperature.

Per serving: Total calories: 316; total fat: 16g; saturated fat: 1g; carbohydrates: 40g; sugar: 6g; fiber: 6g; protein: 8g; sodium: 219mg; cholesterol: 0mg

Mediterranean Couscous Salad

This fresh salad recipe reminds me of a trip I took with my husband to a small Tuscan village in Italy. It was summertime and we had a similar salad as this for lunch on a lovely covered patio. Couscous is a very small type of pasta that cooks quickly and is so tasty. The couscous soaks up the flavors of the lemon juice and olive oil and pairs perfectly with the chopped vegetables.

1¼ cups reduced-sodium vegetable broth

1 cup couscous

1 (15-ounce) can chickpeas, rinsed and drained

1 medium cucumber, peeled and chopped

2 medium tomatoes, chopped

½ cup pitted black olives, chopped

¼ cup fresh flat-leaf parsley, chopped

Juice of 1 lemon

½ teaspoon sea salt

¼ teaspoon freshly ground black pepper

NUT-FREE
DAIRY-FREE
SOY-FREE
VEGAN

Active Time: 15 minutes
Total Time: 30 minutes

Yield: 4 servings
Serving size: 1 cup

TIP: This salad is a great make-ahead recipe. After you make it, divide it into medium food containers with lids. Store in the refrigerator for up to 3 days.

1. Heat the vegetable broth in a medium saucepan over high heat until it comes to a simmer. Turn off the heat but leave the pot on the stove.

2. Add the couscous to the broth, stir, and put the lid on the pot. Let the couscous sit for 5 minutes, or until it has absorbed most of the liquid.

3. Once the couscous is done cooking, remove the lid and use a fork to fluff the couscous. Add the chickpeas, cucumber, tomatoes, olives, parsley, lemon juice, salt, and pepper. Stir to combine.

4. Serve warm, at room temperature, or chilled.

Per serving: Total calories: 319; total fat: 5g; saturated fat: 1g; carbohydrates: 61g; sugar: 6g; fiber: 10g; protein: 13g; sodium: 499mg; cholesterol: 0mg

Shredded Cabbage and Chicken Salad

This healthy salad is full of crunchy texture from the shredded cabbage, with flavors reminiscent of Chinese chicken salad. I skipped the fried noodles that traditionally go on top and used salty crunchy peanuts instead. By using precooked chicken, you can make this salad in about 20 minutes.

3 cups thinly sliced napa cabbage

1 cup shredded carrots

3 cups cooked chicken breast, chopped

3 scallions, sliced

2 tablespoons olive oil

2 tablespoons toasted sesame oil

2 tablespoons reduced-sodium tamari

½ teaspoon dried ginger

¼ teaspoon garlic powder

⅓ cup salted peanuts, chopped

GLUTEN-FREE
DAIRY-FREE
EXTRA QUICK

Active Time: 20 minutes
Total Time: 20 minutes

Yield: 4 servings
Serving size: 1 cup

TIP: If you don't have toasted sesame oil, you can use more olive oil. Also, to save time, you can precook the chicken to use on this salad. Herbed Cubed Chicken (page 153) is a good recipe to use.

1. In a large mixing bowl, combine the cabbage and carrots. Add the chicken and scallions and toss to combine.
2. Put the olive oil, sesame oil, tamari, ginger, and garlic powder in a small mixing bowl. Whisk to mix well.
3. Pour the dressing over the salad and toss to ensure that the dressing is evenly distributed.
4. Top with the peanuts and serve.

Per serving: Total calories: 417; total fat: 28g; saturated fat: 5g; carbohydrates: 8g; sugar: 2g; fiber: 2g; protein: 34g; sodium: 481mg; cholesterol: 79mg

Black Bean and Ground Beef Chili

Chili is traditionally cooked for hours on the stove top, but this quick version using canned beans is just as good. The black beans balance the richness of the meat and make for a healthy, comforting meal. You can serve the chili as is, or top it with a few slices of avocado and salsa for added flavor.

1 pound 85% lean ground beef

1 onion, chopped

2 (15-ounce) cans black beans, rinsed and drained

1 (14.5-ounce) can diced tomatoes, with juices

2 garlic cloves, minced

2 teaspoons chili powder

1 teaspoon ground cumin

½ teaspoon sea salt

½ teaspoon freshly ground black pepper

1 avocado, pitted, peeled, and sliced (optional)

NUT-FREE
GLUTEN-FREE
DAIRY-FREE
SOY-FREE
FREEZER FRIENDLY

Active Time: 15 minutes
Total Time: 25 minutes

Yield: 4 servings
Serving size: 1 cup

1. Heat a large pot over medium heat. Add the beef and onion, sautéing them together for 5 minutes, using a spatula to break up the meat as it cooks.

2. Add the beans, tomatoes, garlic, chili powder, cumin, salt, and pepper to the pot.

3. Reduce the heat to low, cover, and cook for an additional 5 minutes so the beans heat all the way through.

4. Serve it hot, topping with avocado, if desired.

Per serving: Total calories: 474; total fat: 17g; saturated fat: 7g; carbohydrates: 44g; sugar: 7g; fiber: 11g; protein: 36g; sodium: 633mg; cholesterol: 70mg

TIPS: Freeze any leftovers in an airtight container for up to 2 months. Defrost in the refrigerator before reheating in the microwave or on the stove top.

For those who are sensitive to spicy foods, topping the chili with sliced avocado tamps down the heat, much like sour cream does, but is a healthier option.

Coconut–Green Curry Soup with Beef and Vegetables

If you're looking for a warm and comforting Thai-inspired soup full of coconut flavor, then this is the recipe for you. The richness of the steak and coconut milk is nicely balanced with the broccoli and bell pepper. It is mildly spicy from the green curry paste, but not too spicy.

1 tablespoon olive oil

1 pound flank steak, sliced thinly against the grain

3 garlic cloves, minced

1 tablespoon green curry paste

1 (13.5-ounce) can full-fat coconut milk

1 cup reduced-sodium beef broth

1 (12-ounce) bag broccoli florets

1 red bell pepper, sliced

2 tablespoons reduced-sodium tamari

Juice of 1 lime

NUT-FREE
GLUTEN-FREE
DAIRY-FREE

Active Time: 15 minutes
Total Time: 25 minutes

Yield: 4 servings
Serving size: 1 cup

TIP: You can use reduced-fat coconut milk, but I recommend using the full-fat version for the optimal flavor. Look for green curry paste in the Asian section of your grocery store.

1. Heat the oil in a large skillet over medium heat. Add the steak slices and sauté for 2 minutes on each side.

2. Add the garlic and curry paste and cook for an additional 2 minutes.

3. Stir in the coconut milk, beef broth, broccoli, and bell pepper. Let the mixture come up to a simmer, reduce the heat to low, and put a lid on the skillet.

4. Cook, covered, for 5 minutes more. Turn off the heat and stir in the tamari and lime juice.

5. Serve hot.

Per serving: Total calories: 418; total fat: 28g; saturated fat: 16g; carbohydrates: 10g; sugar: 3g; fiber: 2g; protein: 28g; sodium: 627mg; cholesterol: 45mg

Vegetable Minestrone with Penne Pasta

This hearty soup is full of flavor and nutrition and includes both beans and pasta, along with vegetables and Parmesan cheese. It's perfect served right out of the pot, but the leftovers are almost even more delicious when reheated for an easy lunch the next day.

2 tablespoons olive oil

3 carrots, chopped

3 celery stalks, chopped

1 onion, chopped

3 garlic cloves, minced

1 (28-ounce) can diced tomatoes, with juices

1 (15-ounce) can kidney beans, rinsed and drained

4 cups reduced-sodium vegetable broth

2 cups uncooked penne pasta (for gluten-free option, use gluten-free pasta)

½ cup grated Parmesan cheese (omit for vegan option)

NUT-FREE
GLUTEN-FREE
SOY-FREE
VEGAN

Active Time: 10 minutes
Total Time: 25 minutes

Yield: 4 servings
Serving size: 1 cup

1. Pour the olive oil into a large pot set over medium heat. Add the carrots, celery, and onion and sauté for 3 minutes. Stir, then add the garlic and sauté for 1 minute more.

2. Add the tomatoes, beans, broth, and pasta. Turn the heat to high to bring the liquid to a simmer.

3. Once the mixture begins to simmer, reduce the heat to low. Cover the pot, and continue to cook for another 7 minutes, or until the pasta is cooked to al dente.

4. Turn off the heat and stir in the Parmesan cheese. Serve hot.

Per serving: Total calories: 450; total fat: 12g; saturated fat: 3g; carbohydrates: 68g; sugar: 15g; fiber: 11g; protein: 22g; sodium: 1,387mg; cholesterol: 10mg

Curry Chicken and Chickpea Soup

This is a dish for those times when you need delicious comfort. This soup has the familiarity of a traditional chicken soup but with a Moroccan twist, including the chickpeas, spices, and parsley. Serve it with flatbread for an authentic experience.

1 tablespoon olive oil

1 onion, chopped

3 garlic cloves, minced

1 pound boneless, skinless chicken breasts, cut into 1-inch chunks

2 teaspoons curry powder

1 teaspoon ground cumin

1 (15-ounce) can chickpeas, rinsed and drained

1 (15-ounce) can diced tomatoes, with juices

3 cups reduced-sodium chicken broth

2 tablespoons chopped flat-leaf parsley, for topping

NUT-FREE
GLUTEN-FREE
DAIRY-FREE
SOY-FREE
FREEZER FRIENDLY

Active Time: 20 minutes
Total Time: 30 minutes

Yield: 4 servings
Serving size: 1 cup

TIP: Freeze any leftovers in an airtight container for up to 2 months. Defrost in the refrigerator before reheating in the microwave or on the stove top.

1. Heat the olive oil in a large pot over medium heat. Add the onion and garlic and sauté for 3 minutes.

2. Add the chicken, curry powder, and cumin to the pot and stir to combine. Sauté for an additional 5 minutes, stirring occasionally so the chicken starts to cook on all sides.

3. Add the chickpeas, tomatoes, and broth to the pot, turn the heat to high, and bring to a boil.

4. Reduce the heat to low. Cover the pot and continue to cook it for an additional 10 minutes, or until the ingredients have warmed through and the flavors have combined.

5. Serve hot, topped with a sprinkling of chopped fresh parsley.

Per serving: Total calories: 312; total fat: 8g; saturated fat: 1g; carbohydrates: 30g; sugar: 9g; fiber: 7g; protein: 33g; sodium: 867mg; cholesterol: 65mg

Chicken Tortilla Soup

There are so many ways to make this soup, but this one has to be one of the fastest recipes. The chicken is cooked just until tender, and the soup is served with the tortilla chips on the side. If you want even more flavor and richness, you can serve it with sliced avocado on top.

1 tablespoon olive oil

1 onion, chopped

3 garlic cloves, minced

1 pound boneless, skinless chicken breasts, cut into ½-inch chunks

1 teaspoon ground cumin

1 teaspoon chili powder

1 (15-ounce) can chopped tomatoes, with juices

4 cups reduced-sodium chicken broth

1 cup salsa

Tortilla chips, for serving

1 avocado, pitted, peeled, and sliced (optional)

NUT-FREE
GLUTEN-FREE
DAIRY-FREE
SOY-FREE
FREEZER FRIENDLY

Active Time: 20 minutes
Total Time: 27 minutes

Yield: 4 servings
Serving size: 1 cup

1. In a large pot, heat the oil over medium heat.
2. Add the onion and garlic, sautéing them for 2 minutes.
3. Add the chicken, cumin, and chili powder and cook for another 5 minutes, stirring occasionally so the chicken starts to cook on all sides.
4. Add the chopped tomatoes and chicken broth, turn the heat to high, and let the soup come to a boil.
5. Reduce the heat, cover the pot, and cook for an additional 10 minutes, or until all of the ingredients have warmed through.
6. Turn off the heat, stir in the salsa, and serve the soup hot with a side of tortilla chips. Top with avocado, if desired.

TIPS: Freeze any leftovers in an airtight container for up to 2 months. Defrost in the refrigerator before reheating in the microwave or on the stove top.

For those who are sensitive to spicy foods, topping the chili with sliced avocado tamps down the heat, much like sour cream does, but is a healthier option.

Per serving: Total calories: 218; total fat: 7g; saturated fat: 1g; carbohydrates: 15g; sugar: 5g; fiber: 2g; protein: 28g; sodium: 1,236mg; cholesterol: 65mg

Green Chili, Chicken, and White Bean Chili

This chili has lots of spice from the peppers. It can be made in fewer than 30 minutes and is perfect for an easy weeknight meal full of warmth and spice. It can be served as written or topped with avocado slices for an even more Mexican flavor.

1 tablespoon olive oil

1 onion, chopped

3 garlic cloves, minced

1 jalapeño pepper, seeded and chopped

1 pound ground chicken

2 (13.5-ounce) cans white beans, rinsed and drained

1 (4-ounce) can diced green chiles, with juices

2 cups reduced-sodium chicken broth

1 teaspoon ground cumin

1 teaspoon chili powder

¼ teaspoon sea salt

1 avocado, pitted, peeled and sliced (optional)

NUT-FREE
GLUTEN-FREE
DAIRY-FREE
SOY-FREE
FREEZER FRIENDLY

Active Time: 15 minutes

Total Time: 25 minutes

Yield: 4 servings
Serving size: 1 cup

TIPS: Freeze any leftovers in an airtight container for up to 2 months. Defrost in the refrigerator before reheating in the microwave or on the stove top.

For those who are sensitive to spicy foods, topping the chili with sliced avocado tamps down the heat, much like sour cream does, but is a healthier option.

1. In a large pot, heat the olive oil over medium heat.
2. Stir in the onion, garlic, and jalapeño and sauté for 3 minutes.
3. Add the chicken, using a spatula to break up the pieces. Sauté for 3 minutes, or until the chicken is no longer pink.
4. Add the beans, green chiles, chicken broth, cumin, chili powder, and salt. Turn the heat to low and cover the pot.
5. Cook for 5 minutes more, until the beans warm all the way through.
6. Serve hot, topping with sliced avocado, if desired.

Per serving: Total calories: 442; total fat: 17g; saturated fat: 4g; carbohydrates: 37g; sugar: 4g; fiber: 11g; protein: 34g; sodium: 680mg; cholesterol: 95mg

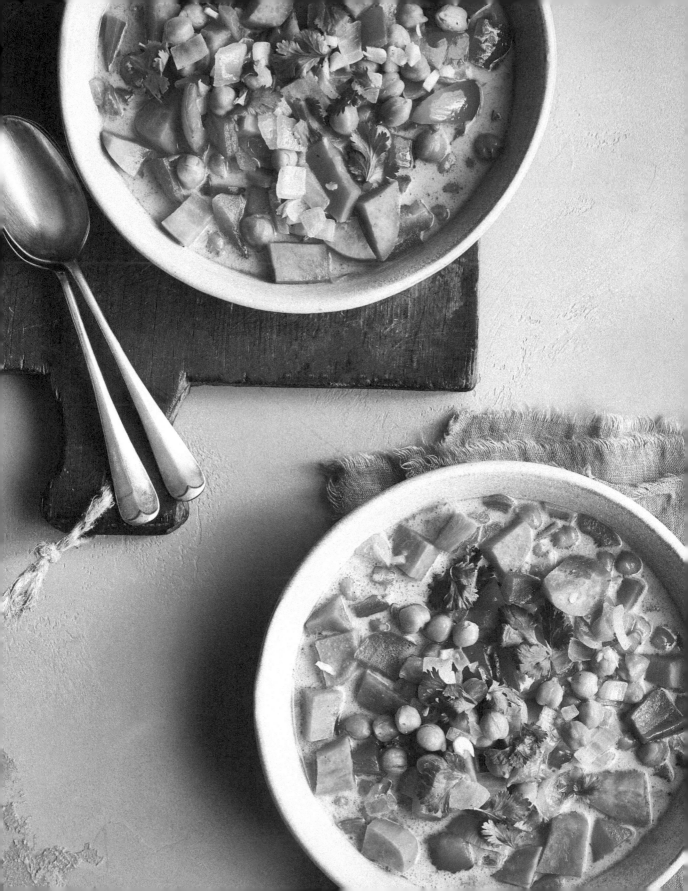

Vegetarian Mains

Sweet Potato and Chickpea Curry Bowls

Sun-Dried Tomato and Hummus Quesadillas

These vegan quesadillas use creamy hummus instead of cheese. Paired with sun-dried tomatoes, they make a healthy and flavorful meal that can be prepared in less than 20 minutes. This three-ingredient recipe is sure to become a family favorite on super busy days.

4 (8-inch) flour tortillas, warmed (for gluten-free option, use gluten-free brown rice tortillas)

⅔ cup prepared hummus

¼ cup drained and chopped sun-dried tomatoes packed in oil

NUT-FREE
GLUTEN-FREE
DAIRY-FREE
SOY-FREE
VEGAN
EXTRA QUICK

Active Time: 10 minutes
Total Time: 20 minutes

Yield: 2 servings
Serving size: 1 quesadilla

1. Lay 2 of the tortillas on a flat surface and spread ⅓ cup of hummus on each.

2. Arrange the sun-dried tomato pieces on top of the hummus. Layer another tortilla on top.

3. Heat a large nonstick skillet over medium heat. Working in two batches, carefully transfer one of the quesdillas into the skillet. Cook for 2 minutes on each side.

4. Remove the quesadilla from the heat and put it on a cutting board.

5. Repeat the previous steps with the remaining quesadilla.

6. Use a knife to cut the quesadillas into wedges. Serve hot or at room temperature.

Per serving: Total calories: 545; total fat: 24g; saturated fat: 5g; carbohydrates: 75g; sugar: 0g; fiber: 8g; protein: 15g; sodium: 961mg; cholesterol: 0mg

Mexican Corn Tortilla and Bean Casserole

I am a huge casserole fan, and I often wonder why I don't make them more often. They're easy to assemble, can be prepared up to several days in advance, and make for wonderful leftovers. This dish is as easy as can be, and it's filled with traditional and lively Mexican flavors. You can use homemade salsa or pico de gallo—your favorite prepared salsa will also do the trick if you're short on time.

Nonstick cooking spray

12 corn tortillas, halved

2 (15-ounce) cans pinto beans, rinsed and drained

1 (16-ounce) jar chunky salsa

3 cups shredded Cheddar cheese

NUT-FREE
GLUTEN-FREE
SOY-FREE
VEGETARIAN
EXTRA QUICK
KIDS LOVE IT

Active Time: 15 minutes
Total Time: 20 minutes

Yield: 6 servings
Serving size: One-sixth of the casserole

1. Preheat the oven to 400°F. Spray a 13-by-9-inch baking dish with nonstick cooking spray and set aside.
2. Arrange half of the corn tortilla halves in the bottom of the baking dish.
3. Pour the beans onto the tortillas and then top the beans with the salsa.
4. Lay the rest of the tortillas on top of the mixture and then layer the cheese on top.
5. Bake the casserole for 20 minutes, or until the cheese is bubbling.
6. Serve hot.

Per serving: Total calories: 474; total fat: 20g; saturated fat: 12g; carbohydrates: 50g; sugar: 3g; fiber: 10g; protein: 24g; sodium: 572mg; cholesterol: 50mg

TIP: Substitute black beans for the pinto beans, if you prefer. To reheat any leftovers, put them on a microwave-safe dish and cover with plastic wrap. Poke a few holes in the wrap and microwave on high for 45 to 60 seconds.

Penne Pasta with Roasted Red Bell Pepper Sauce

For the ultimate in easy but flavorful and healthy meals, try this Penne Pasta with Roasted Red Bell Pepper Sauce. You likely have everything you need to make this dish in your kitchen right now. The red bell pepper sauce is a nice alternative to the usual tomato sauce.

1 (16-ounce) package penne pasta (for gluten-free option, use gluten-free pasta)

1 (16-ounce) jar roasted red bell peppers, drained

⅓ cup olive oil

2 teaspoons balsamic vinegar

1 garlic clove, chopped

1 (4-ounce) package goat cheese, crumbled

NUT-FREE
GLUTEN-FREE
SOY-FREE
VEGETARIAN

Active Time: 15 minutes
Total Time: 25 minutes

Yield: **4 servings**
Serving size: **2 cups**

TIP: You can use feta cheese instead of goat cheese if you prefer.

1. Bring 8 cups of water to a boil in a large pot. Add the pasta and cook it for 10 minutes.

2. While the pasta is cooking, combine the red bell peppers, olive oil, vinegar, and garlic in the pitcher of a blender. Blend on high until the mixture is smooth, stopping occasionally to scrape down the sides of the blender, if necessary.

3. Drain the pasta in a colander once it has fully cooked. Transfer the cooked pasta to a large serving bowl.

4. Pour the sauce over the pasta and toss to combine.

5. Top with the goat cheese and serve warm.

Per serving: Total calories: 666; total fat: 27g; saturated fat: 7g; carbohydrates: 91g; sugar: 5g; fiber: 6g; protein: 20g; sodium: 387mg; cholesterol: 35mg

Vegan Coconut and Mushroom Risotto

This vegan and dairy-free version of risotto uses coconut milk in place of the butter that is traditionally used when making this dish. The result is a creamy rice dish that has the mild aroma and flavor of coconut. The mushrooms add texture and even more flavor.

1 tablespoon olive oil

2 cups chopped mushrooms

1 cup arborio rice

1 (14-ounce) can coconut milk

1 cup reduced-sodium vegetable broth

½ teaspoon sea salt

¼ teaspoon freshly ground black pepper

NUT-FREE
GLUTEN-FREE
DAIRY-FREE
SOY-FREE
VEGAN

Active Time: 15 minutes
Total Time: 30 minutes

1. In a large skillet, heat the olive oil over medium heat. Add the mushrooms and sauté for 3 minutes.
2. Pour the rice into the skillet and stir to mix with the mushrooms.
3. Add the coconut milk and vegetable broth and turn the heat to high. Bring the mixture to a boil and then turn the heat to low.
4. Cover the skillet with a lid and simmer for 20 minutes, or until the rice has absorbed all the liquid.
5. Stir in the salt and pepper and serve hot.

Yield: 4 servings
Serving size: 1 cup

TIP: The best rice to use for this dish is arborio rice, but you can use any short-grain white rice if you can't find arborio rice.

Per serving: Total calories: 378; total fat: 21g; saturated fat: 16g; carbohydrates: 41g; sugar: 3g; fiber: 1g; protein: 5g; sodium: 352mg; cholesterol: 0mg

Crispy Baked Sesame Tofu

This crispy baked tofu is a healthy version of the fried tofu you find in many restaurants. It's a quick and easy way to prepare this plant-based protein, which can be served on top of noodles, with steamed vegetables, or even on its own. Be sure to use extra firm tofu for this recipe, as it won't be necessary to press it before baking.

1 (14-ounce) package extra firm tofu

2 tablespoons cornstarch

2 tablespoons olive oil

½ teaspoon garlic powder

½ teaspoon sea salt

¼ teaspoon freshly ground black pepper

1 tablespoon toasted sesame seeds

NUT-FREE
GLUTEN-FREE
DAIRY-FREE
VEGAN

Active Time: 8 minutes
Total Time: 30 minutes

Yield: 4 servings
Serving size: ½ cup

TIP: To toast the sesame seeds, heat a small non-stick skillet over low heat. Add the sesame seeds and let them toast for about 2 minutes, being careful to not let them burn.

1. Preheat the oven to 400°F. Line a baking sheet with aluminum foil or parchment paper and set aside.

2. Put the tofu on a cutting board and pat it dry with paper towels. Cut the tofu into approximately ½-inch cubes.

3. Transfer the tofu to a large mixing bowl. Add the cornstarch, olive oil, garlic powder, salt, and pepper and toss to combine.

4. Pour the coated tofu pieces onto the baking sheet and spread them out so they aren't touching.

5. Bake the tofu for 20 minutes, flipping the tofu pieces over once during the cooking process. The tofu will turn a golden brown as it cooks.

6. Serve warm or at room temperature, with the toasted sesame seeds sprinkled on top.

Per serving: Total calories: 183; total fat: 13g; saturated fat: 2g; carbohydrates: 8g; sugar: 0g; fiber: 2g; protein: 11g; sodium: 309mg; cholesterol: 0mg

Spicy Black Bean Burgers

These Spicy Black Bean Burgers are a staple in my household. I love using canned beans as the base, since they are so convenient and budget-friendly. You can get creative with how you serve the burgers by placing them on top of a green salad, cooked pasta, or a toasted bun. The spices help jazz up the black beans, making for a tasty plant-based burger that everyone will love.

1 (15-ounce) can black beans, rinsed and drained

1 jalapeño pepper, seeded and finely chopped

½ onion, chopped

2 garlic cloves, minced

½ cup whole wheat bread crumbs

¼ teaspoon chili powder

1 egg, beaten

4 tablespoons olive oil, divided

NUT-FREE
DAIRY-FREE
SOY-FREE
VEGETARIAN
FREEZER FRIENDLY

Active Time: 12 minutes
Total Time: 22 minutes

Yield: 3 servings
Serving size: 1 burger

TIP: You can freeze any leftover cooked burgers in an airtight container or zip-top bag for up to 2 months. Reheat them in the microwave or on the stove top.

1. Pour the black beans into a large mixing bowl. Use the back of a spoon to mash about half of the beans.

2. Add the jalapeño , onion, garlic, bread crumbs, chili powder, egg, and 2 tablespoons of olive oil. Use your hands to mix the ingredients together, and then form 3 burger patties.

3. In a medium skillet, heat the remaining 2 tablespoons of olive oil over medium heat.

4. Add the patties and cover the skillet with a lid. Cook for 5 minutes on each side.

5. Serve hot.

Per serving: Total calories: 513; total fat: 21g; saturated fat: 3g; carbohydrates: 60g; sugar: 5g; fiber: 14g; protein: 21g; sodium: 143mg; cholesterol: 62mg

Shakshuka

Shakshuka is a dish made by cooking eggs in a tomato and red pepper sauce. It has Middle Eastern and North African roots but has become really popular in the United States. Not only is Shakshuka simple to make, but it also has a lovely presentation and is a spicy twist on eggs. My husband loves this dish for lunch served with a piece of flatbread.

1 tablespoon olive oil

½ onion, chopped

1 red bell pepper, cored and chopped

2 garlic cloves, minced

1 (14.5-ounce) can crushed tomatoes, with juices

2 tablespoons tomato paste

¼ teaspoon red pepper flakes

6 eggs

¼ cup crumbled feta cheese

NUT-FREE
GLUTEN-FREE
SOY-FREE
VEGETARIAN
EXTRA QUICK

Active Time: 10 minutes
Total Time: 20 minutes

Yield: 2 servings
Serving size: Half of the dish

TIP: You can leave out the red pepper flakes if you don't like spicy foods.

1. In a large skillet, heat the olive oil over medium heat. Add the onion, bell pepper, and garlic. Sauté for 3 minutes, stirring occasionally.

2. Add the crushed tomatoes, tomato paste, and red pepper flakes and stir to combine.

3. Use a spatula to make a small well in the sauce. Crack an egg into the well.

4. Repeat the previous step five more times, being careful to keep the eggs from touching each other.

5. Reduce the heat to low, cover the skillet, and let cook for 5 minutes, or until the eggs have cooked through.

6. Sprinkle the feta cheese on top and serve hot.

Per serving: Total calories: 405; total fat: 26g; saturated fat: 9g; carbohydrates: 19g; sugar: 9g; fiber: 4g; protein: 30g; sodium: 817mg; cholesterol: 575mg

Vegetarian Pizza Frittata

This baked egg dish might taste a lot like your favorite vegetarian pizza but baked in a fluffy, delicious frittata. This is the perfect easy lunch or dinner when you're craving a pizza but don't have time to make the crust. Simply whisk together the eggs with your favorite toppings and then bake the whole thing until it's ready to be sliced.

1 tablespoon olive oil

½ onion, chopped

½ green bell pepper, chopped

⅓ cup sliced button mushrooms

1 garlic clove, minced

1 teaspoon Italian seasoning

6 eggs, beaten

⅓ cup tomato sauce

1 cup shredded mozzarella cheese, divided

2 tablespoons sliced black olives

NUT-FREE
GLUTEN-FREE
SOY-FREE
VEGETARIAN

Active Time: 10 minutes
Total Time: 30 minutes

Yield: 2 servings
Serving size: Half of the frittata

TIP: If you don't have Italian seasoning, you can use ½ teaspoon dried oregano and ½ teaspoon dried thyme instead.

1. Preheat the oven to 400°F.
2. In a large, oven-safe skillet, heat the oil over medium heat. Add the onion, pepper, mushrooms, garlic, and Italian seasoning and sauté for 3 minutes, stirring occasionally.
3. In a medium mixing bowl, combine the eggs, tomato sauce, and half of the mozzarella cheese. Pour the mixture into the skillet with the vegetables and stir to combine.
4. Allow the egg mixture cook for 2 minutes. Top the mixture with the rest of the cheese and the olives and then carefully transfer the skillet to the oven.
5. Bake for 15 minutes, or until the frittata is completely cooked through. Allow the frittata to cool slightly before slicing and serving.

Per serving: Total calories: 490; total fat: 35g; saturated fat: 13g; carbohydrates: 13g; sugar: 4g; fiber: 2g; protein: 35g; sodium: 790mg; cholesterol: 588mg

Pumpkin Mac and Cheese

For the ultimate in fall-inspired comfort food, try this Pumpkin Mac and Cheese. It's a healthy twist on a comfort food classic, with the addition of canned pumpkin that adds nutrition and fiber without tasting like vegetables. Even kids go crazy for this dish.

---

1 (16-ounce) package elbow pasta

4 tablespoons (½ stick) unsalted butter

¼ cup all-purpose flour

2 cups milk

1 cup canned pumpkin

½ teaspoon mustard powder

½ teaspoon garlic powder

½ teaspoon sea salt

¼ teaspoon freshly ground black pepper

1½ cups shredded Cheddar cheese

NUT-FREE
SOY-FREE
VEGETARIAN
KIDS LOVE IT

Active Time: 15 minutes
Total Time: 25 minutes

Yield: 4 servings
Serving size: 1½ cups

TIP: Look for canned pumpkin with no other ingredients besides pumpkin, especially not pumpkin pie filling (which is a separate product).

1. In a large pot, heat 8 cups of water over high heat. Once the water begins to boil, pour in the pasta and give it a stir.

2. Lower the heat to medium, cover the pot with the lid slightly askew, and allow the pasta to cook for 10 minutes, or for the length of time specified on the package.

3. In a medium saucepan, melt the butter over medium heat while the pasta cooks. Add the flour and whisk until it is well incorporated into the butter.

4. Add the milk, pumpkin, mustard powder, garlic powder, salt, and pepper to the butter-flour mixture. Whisk until fully combined.

5. Add the cheese to the sauce and whisk until smooth. Turn off the heat and cover the saucepan.

6. Drain the cooked pasta in a colander and pour the pasta back into the empty pot.

7. Pour the cheese mixture over the cooked pasta and stir gently to combine. Serve hot.

Per serving: Total calories: 763; total fat: 29g; saturated fat: 17g; carbohydrates: 105g; sugar: 8g; fiber: 5g; protein: 23g; sodium: 625mg; cholesterol: 76mg

Vegan Tempeh Tacos

If you've never had tempeh before, then you're missing out. Made from fermented soybeans, it's a plant-based protein that is mildly nutty in flavor with a terrific firm and chewy texture. These tacos will satisfy both meat-eaters and vegetarians with their spicy and authentic Mexican flavor.

1 tablespoon olive oil

1 onion, chopped

3 garlic cloves, minced

2 (8-ounce) packages tempeh, crumbled

1 cup tomato sauce

½ teaspoon ground cumin

½ teaspoon dried oregano

½ teaspoon sea salt

8 corn tortillas, warmed

2 avocados, pitted, peeled, and sliced

NUT-FREE
GLUTEN-FREE
DAIRY-FREE
VEGAN
EXTRA QUICK

Active Time: 15 minutes
Total Time: 20 minutes

Yield: 4 servings
Serving size: 2 tacos

TIP: You can find tempeh in the refrigerated section of most health-food stores, as well as in the vegan section of many grocery stores.

1. In a large skillet, heat the olive oil over medium heat. Add the onion and garlic and sauté for 5 minutes, stirring occasionally.

2. Add the tempeh, tomato sauce, cumin, oregano, and salt, stirring to combine. Turn the heat to low, cover the skillet, and cook for an additional 5 minutes, until the tempeh warms through fully.

3. When you're ready to serve, put 2 tortillas on each plate. Spoon about ½ cup of the tempeh mixture onto each tortilla and top with a couple of slices of avocado.

4. Serve hot.

Per serving: Total calories: 563; total fat: 30g; saturated fat: 5g; carbohydrates: 55g; sugar: 4g; fiber: 20g; protein: 26g; sodium: 654mg; cholesterol: 0mg

Creamy Quinoa with Artichoke

Artichokes are one of my very favorite vegetables, and they pair perfectly with cooked quinoa and a light dressing of yogurt and lemon juice. The quinoa has a mildly nutty flavor and a chewy texture, and the artichokes are tender and delicious. Even nonvegetarians love this dish.

1 tablespoon olive oil

1 onion, chopped

2 garlic cloves, minced

1 cup quinoa

1¼ cups reduced-sodium vegetable broth

1 (14-ounce) can artichoke hearts, drained and roughly chopped

½ cup reduced-fat Greek yogurt (for vegan option, use dairy-free yogurt)

Juice of 1 lemon

½ teaspoon sea salt

¼ teaspoon freshly ground black pepper

¼ cup toasted pine nuts

GLUTEN-FREE
SOY-FREE
VEGAN

Active Time: 10 minutes
Total Time: 25 minutes

Yield: 4 servings
Serving size: 1 cup

TIP: To toast the pine nuts, put them in a small dry skillet. Turn the heat to low and toast the nuts for about 3 minutes, being careful that they don't burn.

1. In a large saucepan, heat the oil over medium heat. Add the onion and garlic and sauté for 3 minutes, stirring occasionally.

2. Add the quinoa and broth to the pot, turn the heat to high, and to come to a boil.

3. Turn the heat to low, cover the pot, and let the quinoa cook for 12 minutes, or until it has absorbed most of the liquid.

4. Turn off the heat and add the artichokes, yogurt, lemon juice, salt, and pepper, stirring to combine. Top the quinoa with the toasted pine nuts.

5. Serve warm or at room temperature.

Per serving: Total calories: 325; total fat: 13g; saturated fat: 1g; carbohydrates: 44g; sugar: 7g; fiber: 7g; protein: 12g; sodium: 525mg; cholesterol: 4mg

Vegetable Lo Mein

Lo Mein is a traditional Chinese noodle dish. I love this vegetable version that has a quick and easy sauce that kids love. Serve this dish in bowls, along with chopsticks, for the full experience.

1 (10-ounce) package lo mein egg noodles (for gluten-free option, use gluten-free noodles)

1 tablespoon olive oil

3 garlic cloves, minced

1 red bell pepper, sliced into thin strips

2 carrots, julienned

2 cups mushrooms, sliced

1 cup snow peas

2 tablespoons reduced-sodium soy sauce (or tamari for gluten-free option)

1 tablespoon toasted sesame oil

1 teaspoon brown sugar

¼ teaspoon ground ginger

NUT-FREE
GLUTEN-FREE
DAIRY-FREE
VEGETARIAN
KIDS LOVE IT

Active Time: 20 minutes
Total Time: 30 minutes

Yield: 4 servings
Serving size: 1½ cups

TIP: You can use whatever fresh vegetables you have on hand, but you will need a total of about 3 cups of chopped vegetables.

1. In a large pot, bring 8 cups of water to a boil. Add the pasta and cook for 4 minutes, or for the length of time specified on the package. When the noodles have finished cooking, drain in a colander and set aside.

2. In a large skillet, heat the oil over medium heat. Add the garlic, bell pepper, carrots, and mushrooms and sauté for 3 minutes, stirring occasionally.

3. Add the snow peas to the vegetables and cook for 3 minutes more.

4. In a small mixing bowl, whisk together the soy sauce, sesame oil, brown sugar, and ground ginger.

5. In a large mixing bowl, combine the cooked noodles, vegetables, and the sauce. Toss to combine and serve hot.

Per serving: Total calories: 310; total fat: 8g; saturated fat: 2g; carbohydrates: 51g; sugar: 4g; fiber: 4g; protein: 3g; sodium: 1,302mg; cholesterol: 6mg

Tofu Pad Thai

Pad Thai is a traditional dish from Thailand, but it often has a lot of sugar in the sauce. This healthier version has a minimal amount of sugar, but still has tons of flavor from the tamari and fresh lime juice. Don't skip the peanuts on top; they add great crunch and traditional flavor.

1 (8-ounce) package pad thai rice noodles

⅓ cup reduced-sodium tamari

Juice of 4 limes

1 teaspoon Sriracha

2 tablespoons brown sugar

1 tablespoon olive oil

1 (14-ounce) package extra firm tofu, drained and cubed

3 garlic cloves, minced

1 cup shredded carrots

1 cup bean sprouts

⅓ cup peanuts, chopped

GLUTEN-FREE
DAIRY-FREE
VEGAN
KIDS LOVE IT

Active Time: 20 minutes
Total Time: 30 minutes

Yield: 4 servings
Serving size: 1½ cups

TIP: If you don't like spicy food, you can leave out the Sriracha.

1. In a large pot, heat 8 cups of water to a boil. Add the noodles and cook for 5 minutes, or according to the instructions on the package. Drain and rinse, then set aside.

2. In a small mixing bowl, combine the tamari, lime juice, Sriracha, and brown sugar. Whisk to combine, then set aside.

3. In a large skillet, heat the oil over medium heat. Add the tofu and garlic and sauté for 5 minutes, turning the tofu at the halfway point so that it starts to brown on both sides.

4. Add the garlic, carrots, bean sprouts, and cooked rice noodles and stir to combine everything. Pour the sauce over the vegetables and cook for an additional 3 minutes, stirring occasionally.

5. Turn off the heat and top with the peanuts. Serve hot.

Per serving: Total calories: 485; total fat: 16g; saturated fat: 2g; carbohydrates: 71g; sugar: 9g; fiber: 6g; protein: 22g; sodium: 990mg; cholesterol: 0mg

Pineapple Fried Rice

This easy weeknight meal smells heavenly and is always appreciated in my household. This fried rice recipe is low in fat, high in vegetables, and full of tropical pineapple flavor. By using cooked rice in this recipe, you will save a ton of time.

1 tablespoon olive oil

3 carrots, finely chopped

1 red bell pepper, chopped

½ onion, chopped

2 garlic cloves, minced

¼ teaspoon red pepper flakes

2 eggs, lightly beaten

3 cups cooked brown rice

1 (14-ounce) can pineapple chunks, drained

2 tablespoons reduced-sodium tamari

1 teaspoon toasted sesame oil

NUT-FREE
GLUTEN-FREE
DAIRY-FREE
VEGETARIAN
KIDS LOVE IT

Active Time: 15 minutes
Total Time: 23 minutes

Yield: 4 servings
Serving size: 1¼ cups

TIP: You can use cooked white rice instead of the brown rice, if you prefer.

1. In a large skillet, heat the oil over medium heat. Add the carrots, bell pepper, onion, garlic, and red pepper flakes and sauté for 3 minutes.

2. Pour in the eggs and stir to mix them with the vegetables. Sauté for an additional 3 minutes, or until the eggs have fully cooked.

3. Add the rice, pineapple chunks, tamari, and toasted sesame oil, stirring to combine. Cover the pot with a lid and allow to cook for an additional 5 minutes, or until the rice has warmed through.

4. Serve hot.

Per serving: Total calories: 337; total fat: 9g; saturated fat: 2g; carbohydrates: 57g; sugar: 17g; fiber: 6g; protein: 9g; sodium: 421mg; cholesterol: 93mg

Coconut Rice Pilaf with Chickpeas

This hearty rice dish is one of my favorite recipes to make in the middle of the week when time is short, but I want something really flavorful and satisfying. The coconut milk is rich and delicious, and the chickpeas, raisins, and cashews make this pilaf truly outstanding. I think you're going to love this one.

1 tablespoon olive oil

1 onion, chopped

½ teaspoon ground cinnamon

½ teaspoon ground turmeric

1½ cups long-grain white rice

1 cup reduced-sodium vegetable broth

1 (13.5-ounce) can coconut milk

1 (15-ounce) can chickpeas, rinsed and drained

¼ cup golden raisins

¼ cup cashews, chopped

½ teaspoon sea salt

NUT-FREE
GLUTEN-FREE
DAIRY-FREE
SOY-FREE
VEGAN

Active Time: 15 minutes
Total Time: 30 minutes

Yield: 6 servings
Serving size: 1½ cups

TIP: Use regular raisins if you don't have golden raisins on hand.

1. In a large pot, heat the oil over medium heat. Add the onion and sauté for 2 minutes.

2. Add the cinnamon and turmeric, stirring to combine.

3. Pour the rice, broth, and coconut milk into the pot, stirring to combine. Turn the heat to high and let the mixture come to a boil.

4. Turn the heat to low, cover the pot, and let the rice cook for 20 minutes.

5. Turn off the heat once the rice has finished cooking. Remove the lid and use a fork to fluff the rice.

6. Add the chickpeas, raisins, cashews, and salt and stir one last time to combine.

7. Serve hot.

Per serving: Total calories: 438; total fat: 18g; saturated fat: 11g; carbohydrates: 60g; sugar: 8g; fiber: 6g; protein: 9g; sodium: 239mg; cholesterol: 0mg

Sweet Potato and Chickpea Curry Bowls

This curry is a hearty and flavorful stew that can be served right out of the pot or with a side of steamed rice. It's full of nourishing vegetables in a creamy coconut milk base. Even kids like this one because it's not too spicy.

1 tablespoon olive oil

1 onion, chopped

1 red bell pepper, chopped

3 garlic cloves, minced

2 sweet potatoes, cubed

1 (15-ounce) can chickpeas, rinsed and drained

1 cup reduced-sodium vegetable broth

1 (13.5-ounce) can coconut milk

1 tablespoon curry powder

¼ teaspoon ground ginger

½ teaspoon sea salt

¼ teaspoon freshly ground black pepper

NUT-FREE
GLUTEN-FREE
DAIRY-FREE
SOY-FREE
VEGAN
KIDS LOVE IT
FREEZER FRIENDLY

Active Time: 13 minutes
Total Time: 30 minutes

Yield: 4 servings
Serving size: 1½ cups

TIP: You can freeze leftovers in an airtight container for up to 2 months. Reheat in the microwave or on the stove top.

1. In a large pot, heat the olive oil over medium heat. Add the onion, bell pepper, and garlic and sauté for 3 minutes, stirring occasionally.

2. Add the sweet potatoes, chickpeas, broth, coconut milk, curry powder, and ground ginger and stir to combine. Turn the heat to high and bring the pot to a boil.

3. Turn the heat to low, cover the pot, and cook for 18 minutes, or until the sweet potato is fork-tender.

4. Stir in the salt and pepper and serve hot.

Per serving: Total calories: 427; total fat: 24g; saturated fat: 16g; carbohydrates: 46g; sugar: 10g; fiber: 10g; protein: 10g; sodium: 367mg; cholesterol: 0mg

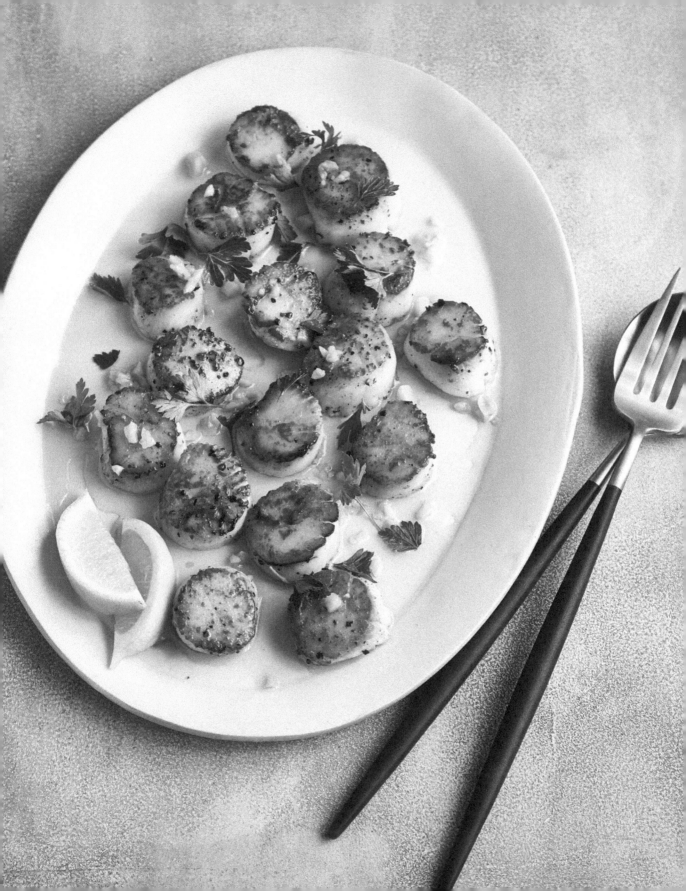

Seafood

Scallops with Lemon-Butter Sauce

Chipotle-Baked Salmon

Baked salmon is one of those back-pocket recipes that you can use when you have an extra-busy day. I love this recipe because it requires minimal preparation and the oven does all the work while you unwind or catch up on chores around the house. The mayonnaise topping offers a nice balance of spiciness and creaminess and goes really well with the meaty salmon fillets.

4 salmon fillets

⅓ cup mayonnaise

2 teaspoons ground chipotle powder

¼ teaspoon garlic powder

½ teaspoon sea salt

¼ teaspoon freshly ground black pepper

NUT-FREE
GLUTEN-FREE
DAIRY-FREE
SOY-FREE

Active Time: 10 minutes
Total Time: 25 minutes

Yield: 4 servings
Serving size: 1 fillet

TIP: Halibut or mahi-mahi work just as well as salmon for this recipe.

1. Preheat the oven to 375°F. Line a baking sheet with parchment paper.

2. Lay the salmon fillets on the baking sheet, skin-side down.

3. In a small mixing bowl, combine the mayonnaise, chipotle powder, garlic powder, salt, and pepper.

4. Use a spoon to divide the mixture between the salmon fillets. Gently spread the mayonnaise mixture on the top of each fillet.

5. Bake the salmon for 17 minutes, or until a meat thermometer inserted into the thickest part of the fish reaches 140°F. Serve hot.

Per serving: Total calories: 300; total fat: 23g; saturated fat: 4g; carbohydrates: <1g; sugar: 2g; fiber: <1g; protein: 23g; sodium: 448mg; cholesterol: 50mg

Parmesan and Tomato Foil-Baked Halibut

Cooking fish in foil packets is one of my favorite tips to keep the fillets moist and tender and save time cleaning up later. The packets lock in all the delicious flavors from the tomato and cheese. I like to serve the cooked halibut with a pasta salad or steamed rice.

4 halibut fillets

½ teaspoon sea salt

¼ teaspoon freshly ground black pepper

4 fresh tomato slices

4 tablespoons freshly grated Parmesan cheese

1 lemon, cut into wedges

NUT-FREE
GLUTEN-FREE
SOY-FREE

Active Time: 10 minutes
Total Time: 25 minutes

Yield: **4 servings**
Serving size: **1 fillet**

TIP: You can substitute mahi-mahi or salmon for the halibut.

1. Preheat the oven to 400°F. Tear off four 14-inch lengths of aluminum foil for the packets and lay them on a flat surface.

2. Pat the fillets dry with a paper towel. Place each fillet on the lower half of each piece of aluminum foil.

3. Sprinkle the salt and pepper on the fillets.

4. Top each fillet with a tomato slice and 1 tablespoon of cheese.

5. Fold the foil over the top of the fish and seal the edges.

6. Put the foil packets on a baking sheet and bake for 15 minutes.

7. Open each packet carefully and serve hot, with a wedge of fresh lemon.

Per serving: Total calories: 196; total fat: 4g; saturated fat: 1g; carbohydrates: 2g; sugar: 1g; fiber: <1g; protein: 34g; sodium: 496mg; cholesterol: 47mg

Panfried Tilapia with White Wine Sauce

This panfried tilapia topped with a butter and wine sauce is a surprisingly easy way to serve a gourmet dinner. Tilapia is a neutral-tasting white fish that is flaky and light. This dish is great served with a side of steamed vegetables and rice.

2 tablespoons olive oil

4 tilapia fillets

½ teaspoon sea salt

¼ teaspoon freshly ground black pepper

3 tablespoons unsalted butter

2 garlic cloves, minced

¾ cup white wine

NUT-FREE
GLUTEN-FREE
SOY-FREE

Active Time: 12 minutes

Total Time: 22 minutes

Yield: 4 servings
Serving size: 1 fillet

TIP: Mahi-mahi or halibut work just as well as tilapia for this recipe.

1. In a large skillet, heat the olive oil over medium heat. Add the fish and cook it for 4 minutes. Season the fillets with the salt and pepper.

2. Turn the fish over and cook for an additional 3 minutes. Remove the fish to a serving plate and cover with foil to keep warm.

3. Put the butter in the skillet and allow to melt. Add the garlic and sauté for 2 minutes.

4. Pour in the white wine and let it cook for 2 minutes. Turn off the heat and pour the sauce over the fish. Serve hot.

Per serving: Total calories: 268; total fat: 17g; saturated fat: 7g; carbohydrates: 1g; sugar: 0g; fiber: 1g; protein: 23g; sodium: 535mg; cholesterol: 73mg

Scallops with Lemon-Butter Sauce

A type of shellfish, scallops are one of my favorite foods. They are neutral in flavor and are simply divine with this lemon-butter sauce. For the ultimate in easy meals, try this dish served with steamed asparagus and a baked potato.

2 tablespoons olive oil

1 pound scallops (about 16 large scallops)

½ teaspoon sea salt

¼ teaspoon freshly ground black pepper

3 tablespoons unsalted butter

2 garlic cloves, minced

Juice of 1 lemon

NUT-FREE
GLUTEN-FREE
SOY-FREE

Active Time: 12 minutes
Total Time: 22 minutes

Yield: 4 servings
Serving size: 4 scallops

TIP: You can buy scallops frozen in most grocery stores. Just defrost them in the refrigerator overnight before preparing.

1. In a large skillet, heat the olive oil over medium-high heat. Season the scallops with the salt and pepper.

2. Add the scallops to the skillet and cook for 3 minutes per side. Transfer the scallops to a serving plate and cover with foil to keep warm.

3. Turn the heat to low, put the butter in the skillet, and let it melt. Add the garlic and sauté for 2 minutes.

4. Turn off the heat, stir in the lemon juice, and pour the sauce over the scallops. Serve hot.

Per serving: Total calories: 242; total fat: 17g; saturated fat: 7g; carbohydrates: 4g; sugar: <1g; fiber: <1g; protein: 19g; sodium: 535mg; cholesterol: 61mg

Sheet Pan Teriyaki Halibut and Snow Peas

Sheet pan meals are those for which you put all of your ingredients on a baking sheet and everything gets cooked together for the same amount of time. This is a great technique for quick and easy meals and works really well with this dish. The fish is flavorful and tender, and the snow peas are crisp and fresh.

2 tablespoons brown sugar

½ teaspoon garlic powder

¼ cup reduced-sodium tamari

¼ teaspoon ground ginger

4 halibut fillets

2 cups fresh snow peas

1 medium onion, chopped

NUT-FREE
GLUTEN-FREE
DAIRY-FREE

Active Time: 10 minutes
Total Time: 30 minutes

1. Preheat the oven to 400°F. Line a baking sheet with parchment paper and set aside.

2. In a small mixing bowl, combine the brown sugar, 2 tablespoons of water, the garlic powder, tamari, and ground ginger. Whisk until fully mixed.

3. In a large bowl, combine the halibut, snow peas, and onion. Pour the sauce over the ingredients and toss gently to combine them.

4. Arrange the fish and vegetables on the sheet pan. Bake for 20 minutes, or until the fish is cooked all the way through.

5. Serve hot.

Yield: 4 servings
Serving size: 1 fillet

TIP: You can substitute salmon for the halibut in this recipe.

Per serving: Total calories: 219; total fat: 4g; saturated fat: 1g; carbohydrates: 13g; sugar: 7g; fiber: 2g; protein: 34g; sodium: 957mg; cholesterol: 47mg

Tuna Patties with Chipotle Mayo

Canned tuna makes a great base for these delicious tuna patties served with a spicy chipotle mayo topping. Almond flour keeps this recipe gluten-free and adds a little bit of texture to the patties. I like to serve these alongside a simple green salad and cooked quinoa.

2 (5-ounce) cans
tuna, drained

1 egg

¼ cup almond flour

¼ teaspoon garlic powder

2 tablespoons olive oil,
divided

½ cup mayonnaise

¼ teaspoon
chipotle powder

Juice of 1 lemon

GLUTEN-FREE
DAIRY-FREE
SOY-FREE
EXTRA QUICK

Active Time: 10 minutes
Total Time: 20 minutes

Yield: 4 servings
Serving size: 1 patty

TIP: Look for a quality brand of tuna. I like to use albacore tuna that is canned without any oil or salt. For an interesting variation on this recipe, try using canned salmon in place of the tuna.

1. In a medium bowl, combine the tuna, egg, almond flour, garlic powder, and 1 tablespoon of olive oil. Use a fork to combine the ingredients, and then use your hands to form 4 patties.

2. In a medium skillet, heat the remaining 1 tablespoon of olive oil over medium heat. Add the patties and cook for 4 minutes on each side.

3. In a small mixing bowl, combine the mayonnaise, chipotle powder, and lemon juice while the patties cook. Stir to combine.

4. Serve the tuna patties with a dollop of the mayonnaise, hot or at room temperature.

Per serving: Total calories: 361; total fat: 33g; saturated fat: 5g; carbohydrates: 3g; sugar: 4g; fiber: 1g; protein: 16g; sodium: 298mg; cholesterol: 79mg

Skillet-Cooked Shrimp and Asparagus with Lemon

Tender shrimp and buttery asparagus make the perfect match in this easy skillet dish. The lemon juice adds brightness to the fish and the vegetables, and a hint of garlic adds pop. Serve it plain or on top of steamed rice for a satisfying meal.

2 tablespoons olive oil

2 garlic cloves, minced

1 pound shrimp, peeled and deveined

½ teaspoon sea salt

¼ teaspoon freshly ground black pepper

2 tablespoons unsalted butter

1 pound asparagus, cut into 3-inch pieces

Juice of 2 lemons

NUT-FREE
GLUTEN-FREE
SOY-FREE

Active Time: 15 minutes
Total Time: 25 minutes

Yield: 4 servings
Serving size: One-quarter of the dish

TIP: If you can't find fresh asparagus, you can find it frozen, but you will need to add 5 minutes to the cooking time.

1. In a large skillet, heat the olive oil over medium heat. Add the garlic and sauté for 2 minutes.

2. Add the shrimp to the skillet and season with the salt and pepper. Cook the shrimp for 3 minutes on each side.

3. Remove the shrimp to a serving plate and cover with foil to keep warm.

4. Put the butter in the skillet and let it melt. Add the asparagus and cook for 4 minutes.

5. Turn off the heat and pour the lemon juice over the asparagus.

6. Transfer the asparagus to the serving plate and toss gently with the shrimp. Serve hot.

Per serving: Total calories: 252; total fat: 14g; saturated fat: 5g; carbohydrates: 8g; sugar: 3g; fiber: 3g; protein: 27g; sodium: 588mg; cholesterol: 222mg

Tuna-Stuffed Avocados

Almost everyone loves tuna salad, and this lower-carb recipe combines my favorite tuna salad recipe with the creaminess of ripe avocado. This satisfying meal also makes for a great snack. Just a grab a spoon and dig in.

2 (5-ounce) cans tuna, drained

½ cup mayonnaise

2 tablespoons pickle relish

1 teaspoon Dijon mustard

2 celery stalks, chopped

¼ onion, chopped

¼ teaspoon sea salt

¼ teaspoon freshly ground black pepper

4 small-to-medium avocados, pitted

NUT-FREE
GLUTEN-FREE
DAIRY-FREE
SOY-FREE
EXTRA QUICK

Active Time: 10 minutes

Total Time: 15 minutes

1. In a medium mixing bowl, combine the tuna, mayonnaise, relish, mustard, celery, onion, salt, and pepper. Stir to combine.

2. Cut the avocados in half lengthwise and remove the pit but leave the peel. Use a spoon to fill each hollow of the avocado with tuna salad. Serve immediately.

Yield: 4 servings
Serving size: 2 avocado halves

TIP: If you don't plan to serve this right away, wait to cut the avocados until just before eating.

Per serving: Total calories: 400; total fat: 34g; saturated fat: 5g; carbohydrates: 12g; sugar: 6g; fiber: 7g; protein: 15g; sodium: 551mg; cholesterol: 33mg

Pesto-Baked Salmon and Vegetables

This is the perfect dish for any time when fresh basil is plentiful as it makes an easy homemade pesto for the salmon and vegetables. This is another sheet pan dinner that can be served on a weeknight or at a dinner party. I like to plate the fish with a scoop of steamed white or brown rice on the side.

4 salmon fillets

⅓ cup olive oil

1 cup fresh basil leaves

⅓ cup pine nuts

2 garlic cloves, minced

½ teaspoon sea salt

¼ teaspoon freshly ground black pepper

2 cups broccoli florets

1 sweet potato, thinly sliced

GLUTEN-FREE
DAIRY-FREE
SOY-FREE

Active Time: 10 minutes
Total Time: 30 minutes

Yield: 4 servings
Serving size: 1 fillet

TIP: You can substitute halibut or mahi-mahi for the salmon.

1. Preheat the oven to 400°F. Line a baking sheet with parchment paper.

2. Lay the salmon on the baking sheet, skin-side down.

3. Make the pesto by combining the olive oil, basil, pine nuts, garlic, salt, and pepper in the pitcher of a food processor or blender. Process or blend on high until the pesto is smooth.

4. Use a spoon to divide half of the pesto between the salmon fillets, using the back of the spoon to spread it around.

5. In a medium mixing bowl, combine the broccoli florets and the sweet potato. Add the rest of the pesto and toss to combine. Arrange the vegetables on the baking sheet with the salmon.

6. Bake for 15 minutes, or until a meat thermometer inserted into the thickest part of the fish reaches 140°F. Serve hot.

Per serving: Total calories: 428; total fat: 30g; saturated fat: 4g; carbohydrates: 12g; sugar: 3g; fiber: 3g; protein: 26g; sodium: 361mg; cholesterol: 85mg

Shrimp Scampi with Zucchini Noodles

This updated version of shrimp scampi uses healthy and delicious zucchini noodles in place of traditional pasta. The flavors are the same, but the dish feels lighter and fresher with the zucchini. The sprinkle of Parmesan cheese at the end just brings it all together into a wonderful meal.

2 tablespoons olive oil

2 garlic cloves, minced

1 pound shrimp, peeled and deveined

½ teaspoon sea salt

¼ teaspoon freshly ground black pepper

¼ teaspoon red pepper flakes

2 tablespoons unsalted butter

2 large zucchini, spiralized

Juice of 1 lemon

2 tablespoons grated Parmesan cheese

NUT-FREE
GLUTEN-FREE
SOY-FREE

Active Time: 20 minutes
Total Time: 30 minutes

Yield: 4 servings
Serving size: One-quarter of the dish

TIP: If you don't have a spiralizer, you can use a cheese grater or a vegetable peeler to make the zucchini noodles. Some grocery stores also sell zucchini noodles in the produce section.

1. In a large skillet, heat the olive oil over medium heat. Add the garlic and sauté for 2 minutes.

2. Add the shrimp to the skillet and season with the salt and pepper. Cook for 3 minutes on each side.

3. Transfer the shrimp to a serving plate and cover with foil to keep warm.

4. Put the butter in the skillet, allowing it to melt. Add the zucchini noodles and cook for 3 minutes, stirring often.

5. Turn off the heat and put the cooked shrimp back into the skillet with the noodles. Pour the lemon juice over the top and toss to combine. Sprinkle the cheese over the top and serve hot.

Per serving: Total calories: 236; total fat: 15g; saturated fat: 5g; carbohydrates: 10g; sugar: 3g; fiber: 3g; protein: 22g; sodium: 510mg; cholesterol: 163mg

Kung Pao Shrimp

This dish is traditionally quite spicy. However, while this version is full of flavor, it's not so spicy that kids won't eat it. I like to serve this easy shrimp dinner over steamed white rice.

¼ cup reduced-sodium soy sauce or tamari

2 tablespoons honey

2 teaspoons cornstarch

1 teaspoon chili paste

1 teaspoon rice wine vinegar

½ teaspoon ground ginger

2 tablespoons olive oil

1 pound shrimp, peeled and deveined

1 red bell pepper, sliced

¼ cup chopped peanuts

DAIRY-FREE

Active Time: 20 minutes
Total Time: 30 minutes

Yield: **4 servings**
Serving size: **One-quarter of the dish**

TIP: Don't leave out the cornstarch, as it helps thicken the sauce.

1. In a medium bowl or pitcher, whisk together the soy sauce, honey, 2 tablespoons of water, the cornstarch, chili paste, vinegar, and ginger. Set aside.

2. In a large skillet, heat the olive oil over medium heat.

3. Add the shrimp and bell pepper to the skillet and cook for 3 minutes. Turn the shrimp over and pour in the sauce.

4. Cook the shrimp and sauce for 5 minutes, stirring occasionally.

5. Turn off the heat and sprinkle in the peanuts. Serve hot.

Per serving: Total calories: 255; total fat: 13g; saturated fat: 2g; carbohydrates: 15g; sugar: 10g; fiber: 1g; protein: 23g; sodium: 872mg; cholesterol: 145mg

Tuna Melt

The next time you crave a tuna melt, give this recipe a try. It can be made in just about 20 minutes and is great served with a green salad or fresh, sliced tomatoes. Nobody will complain about having these delicious sandwiches for dinner.

2 (5-ounce) cans tuna, drained

2 celery stalks, chopped

¼ cup mayonnaise

2 tablespoons pickle relish

1 teaspoon Dijon mustard

¼ onion, chopped

¼ teaspoon sea salt

¼ teaspoon freshly ground black pepper

8 slices bread (for gluten-free option, use gluten-free bread)

4 slices provolone cheese

Nonstick cooking spray

NUT-FREE
GLUTEN-FREE
SOY-FREE
EXTRA QUICK

Active Time: 10 minutes
Total Time: 20 minutes

Yield: 4 servings
Serving size: 1 sandwich

TIP: Try using Cheddar cheese instead of provolone for a sharper, brighter flavor.

1. In a medium mixing bowl, combine the tuna, celery, mayonnaise, relish, mustard, onion, salt, and pepper. Stir well and set aside.

2. Put 4 slices of bread on a flat surface. Spoon the tuna salad onto the bread slices and top with a slice of cheese. Place the remaining pieces of bread on the top of the cheese to make a sandwich.

3. Spray the surface of a large nonstick skillet with nonstick cooking spray and heat over medium heat. Toast each sandwich on the skillet for 2 minutes.

4. Turn the sandwiches over and toast for 3 minutes more, or until the cheese starts to melt. Serve hot.

Per serving: Total calories: 403; total fat: 21g; saturated fat: 7g; carbohydrates: 32g; sugar: 8g; fiber: 4g; protein: 25g; sodium: 1,001mg; cholesterol: 48mg

Easy Fish Tacos

In California, people line up at the best beach shacks for fresh fish tacos. I've re-created the experience with this easy recipe, using a neutral white fish, spicy seasoning, and a crunchy topping of shredded cabbage and onions. Finishing it with sliced avocado helps balance the chili powder, making for a fish taco that is out of this world.

2 tablespoons olive oil

4 tilapia fillets, cut in half

1 teaspoon chili powder

½ teaspoon smoked paprika

½ teaspoon sea salt

¼ teaspoon freshly ground black pepper

12 corn tortillas, warmed

½ small purple cabbage, shredded

½ onion, diced

1 avocado, pitted, peeled, and sliced

2 limes, halved

NUT-FREE
GLUTEN-FREE
SOY-FREE

Active Time: 12 minutes
Total Time: 22 minutes

Yield: 6 servings
Serving size: 2 tacos

TIP: You can use whatever whitefish you prefer, including halibut or mahi-mahi.

1. In a large skillet, heat the olive oil over medium heat.
2. Season the fish with the chili powder, paprika, salt, and pepper.
3. Put the seasoned fish in the skillet and cook for 3 minutes per side, until cooked fully.
4. Divide the fish fillets between the tortillas.
5. Top each taco with cabbage, onion, slice of avocado, and a squeeze of fresh lime juice. Serve hot.

Per serving: Total calories: 493; total fat: 19g; saturated fat: 3g; carbohydrates: 67g; sugar: 8g; fiber: 16g; protein: 28g; sodium: 390mg; cholesterol: 55mg

Garlic Noodles with Shrimp

You can't go wrong with a hot, flavorful noodle dish when you're craving comfort food. This one is rich in garlic flavor balanced with tender noodles and vegetables. This is one of those dishes that you'll want to make over and over again.

1 (12-ounce) package spaghetti (for gluten-free option, use gluten-free pasta)

2 tablespoons olive oil, divided

1 pound shrimp, peeled and deveined

2 carrots, sliced

1 red bell pepper, thinly sliced

½ onion, sliced

4 garlic cloves, minced

⅓ cup reduced-sodium soy sauce or tamari

2 tablespoons rice vinegar

1 tablespoon brown sugar

½ teaspoon ground ginger

NUT-FREE
GLUTEN-FREE
DAIRY-FREE

Active Time: 20 minutes
Total Time: 30 minutes

Yield: 4 servings
Serving size: 1 cup

1. In a large pot, bring 8 cups of water to a boil. Add the pasta and cook for 10 minutes.

2. While the pasta cooks, heat 1 tablespoon of oil in a large skillet. Add the shrimp, cooking for 3 minutes on each side, until the shrimp have turned pink.

3. Transfer the cooked shrimp to a serving plate.

4. Heat the remaining 1 tablespoon of oil in the skillet. Add the carrots, bell pepper, onion, and garlic. Sauté the vegetables for 4 minutes, stirring occasionally.

CONTINUED

5. In a small mixing bowl, combine the soy sauce, vinegar, brown sugar, and ginger, whisking to combine. Drain the pasta in a colander once it has fully cooked. Transfer the cooked pasta to a large serving bowl.

6. Pour the sauce, cooked shrimp, and vegetables over the pasta and toss to combine.

7. Serve hot.

Per serving: Total calories: 515; total fat: 10g; saturated fat: 1g; carbohydrates: 76g; sugar: 7g; fiber: 4g; protein: 32g; sodium: 1,020mg; cholesterol: 145mg

Coconut Shrimp Curry

Shrimp is great for a quick meal because it cooks really fast. The base of this curry includes tomatoes and coconut milk, making this a really hearty and flavorful dish. The curry powder adds even more flavor without being overly spicy, and the scent is heavenly.

2 tablespoons olive oil

1 onion, chopped

2 garlic cloves, minced

2 carrots, julienned

2 teaspoons curry powder

½ teaspoon sea salt

¼ teaspoon freshly ground black pepper

1 (14.5-ounce) can diced tomatoes, with juices

1 (13.5-ounce) can coconut milk

1 pound shrimp, peeled and deveined

Juice of 1 lemon

2 scallions, sliced

NUT-FREE
GLUTEN-FREE
DAIRY-FREE
SOY-FREE

Active Time: 15 minutes

Total Time: 25 minutes

Yield: 4 servings
Serving size: 1 cup

1. In a large saucepan, heat the oil over medium heat. Add the onion and garlic and sauté for 3 minutes.

2. Add the carrots, curry powder, salt, and pepper, stirring to combine.

3. Gently drop in the tomatoes, turn the heat to high, and stir to combine. Allow the mixture to come to a simmer.

4. Add the coconut milk and shrimp, turn the heat to low, and cover the pot. Let cook for 8 minutes.

5. Turn off the heat and stir in the lemon juice. Top with the sliced scallions.

6. Serve hot.

Per serving: Total calories: 371; total fat: 26g; saturated fat: 16g; carbohydrates: 17g; sugar: 8g; fiber: 3g; protein: 21g; sodium: 716mg; cholesterol: 145mg

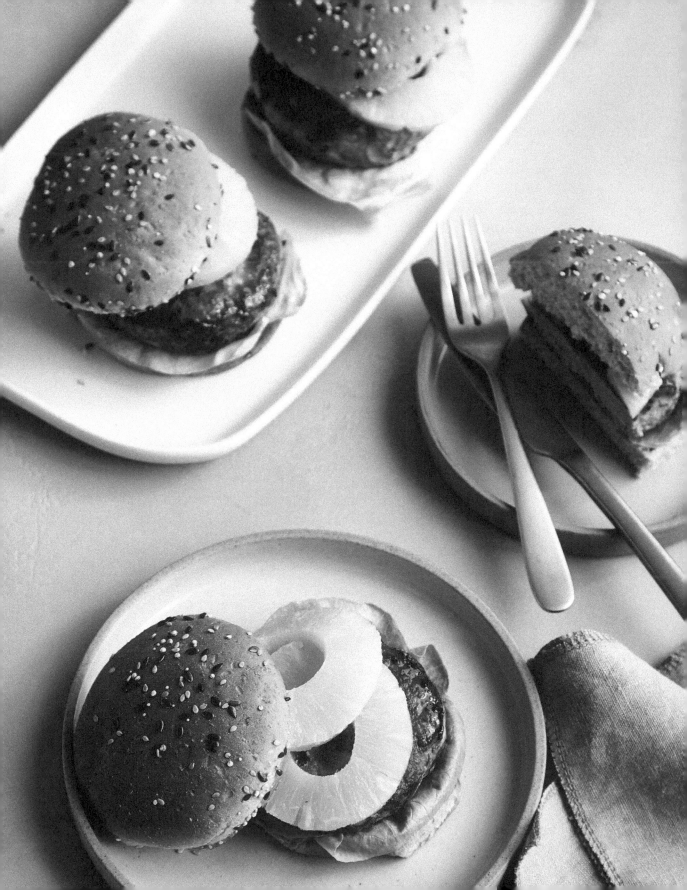

Poultry

Pineapple Turkey Burgers

Healthy Baked Chicken Nuggets

This healthier version of chicken nuggets uses whole wheat flour for the breading. It also uses the meat from chicken breasts, as opposed to processed pieces of chicken. The nuggets are baked as opposed to fried, making these a healthy alternative to traditional nuggets. I like to serve them with baked sweet potato fries or my Cinnamon-Roasted Butternut Squash (page 121) for the ultimate healthy comfort food meal.

4 boneless, skinless chicken breasts, cut lengthwise into 1-inch slices

3 eggs

1 cup whole wheat bread crumbs (for gluten-free option, use gluten-free bread crumbs)

½ teaspoon sea salt

¼ teaspoon freshly ground black pepper

NUT-FREE
GLUTEN-FREE
DAIRY-FREE
SOY-FREE
KIDS LOVE IT

Active Time: 10 minutes
Total Time: 30 minutes

Yield: 4 servings
Serving size: One-quarter of the nuggets

TIP: You can find whole wheat or gluten-free bread crumbs in the baking aisle of most grocery stores.

1. Preheat the oven to 425°F. Line a baking sheet with parchment paper and set aside.

2. In a small bowl, beat the eggs. Put the bread crumbs on a plate.

3. Working one slice at a time, dip the chicken into the egg mixture. Shake off the excess egg and then dip the chicken into the bread crumbs.

4. Lay the breaded chicken slices on the baking sheet, leaving room between each piece.

5. Bake the chicken for 20 minutes flipping them over halfway through.

6. Sprinkle with the salt and pepper and serve hot.

Per serving: Total calories: 255; total fat: 7g; saturated fat: 2g; carbohydrates: 16g; sugar: 2g; fiber: 2g; protein: 31g; sodium: 698mg; cholesterol: 205mg

Chicken and Feta Cheese Pasta

This dish has traditional Mediterranean flavors, including feta cheese, tomatoes, basil, and lemon. I like to serve this dish hot the day I make it and then serve the leftovers chilled the next day for lunch. Don't forget the freshly squeezed lemon juice to help brighten up this delightful pasta dish.

1 (16-ounce) package bow-tie pasta, also known as farfalle (for gluten-free option, use gluten-free pasta)

2 tablespoons olive oil

2 boneless, skinless chicken breasts, chopped into bite-size pieces

1 cup cherry tomatoes, halved

4 ounces feta cheese, crumbled

8 basil leaves, chopped

2 lemons, juiced

NUT-FREE
GLUTEN-FREE
SOY-FREE

Active Time: 20 minutes

Total Time: 30 minutes

Yield: 4 servings
Serving size: 1½ cups

TIP: If you don't have fresh basil, you can use 1 teaspoon of dried basil leaves instead.

1. In a large pot, heat 8 cups of water over high heat. Once the water comes to a boil, pour in the pasta and give it a stir.

2. Lower the heat to medium, cover the pot with the lid slightly askew, and let the pasta cook for 10 minutes, or according to the package instructions.

3. In a medium saucepan, heat the oil over medium heat while the pasta cooks.

4. Add the chicken and cook for 12 minutes, stirring occasionally so the chicken cooks evenly on all sides.

5. Turn off the heat and add the tomatoes to the chicken, stirring to combine.

6. Drain the cooked pasta in a colander and pour the pasta back into the empty pot.

7. Pour the chicken and tomato mixture over the pasta and toss to combine.

8. Top the pasta with the feta cheese, basil, and lemon juice. Stir once more before serving hot.

Per serving: Total calories: 604; total fat: 16g; saturated fat: 6g; carbohydrates: 89g; sugar: 5g; fiber: 5g; protein: 30g; sodium: 410mg; cholesterol: 58mg

Lightened-Up Chicken Parmesan

This healthier version of Chicken Parmesan is baked in the oven instead of fried. I promise you are going to be very happy with the crispy breading. I like to serve this dish with a salad or green vegetable on the side.

4 boneless, skinless chicken breasts

½ cup whole wheat bread crumbs

½ cup grated Parmesan cheese

2 eggs

Nonstick cooking spray

1 cup marinara sauce

½ cup shredded mozzarella cheese

NUT-FREE
SOY-FREE
KIDS LOVE IT

Active Time: 15 minutes
Total Time: 30 minutes

Yield: 4 servings
Serving size: 2 pieces

1. Preheat the oven to 425°F. Line a baking sheet with parchment paper and set aside.
2. Use a sharp knife to cut each chicken breast in half lengthwise. Lay the chicken slices on a cutting board and cover with a piece of plastic wrap. Use a mallet to pound them flat.
3. In a small mixing bowl, stir together the bread crumbs and Parmesan cheese.
4. Beat the eggs in another small mixing bowl.
5. Dunk each piece of chicken in the egg mixture and then into the bread crumb mixture. Put the chicken on the baking sheet.

6. Lightly spray the tops of the chicken pieces with nonstick cooking spray to help them brown in the oven.

7. Bake the chicken for 12 minutes, until nicely browned.

8. Remove the chicken from the oven and top with the marinara sauce and mozzarella cheese.

9. Return the chicken to the oven for another 3 minutes so the cheese can melt.

10. Serve hot.

Per serving: Total calories: 324; total fat: 13g; saturated fat: 5g; carbohydrates: 14g; sugar: 4g; fiber: 2g; protein: 38g; sodium: 878mg; cholesterol: 175mg

Lemon Chicken with Couscous

My husband and I went on a Mediterranean cruise for our honeymoon over fifteen years ago; this dish reminds me of the food we enjoyed on that trip. The chicken is tender and flavorful, and goes perfectly with the lemon-infused couscous. Fresh parsley and pickled onions add extra texture and brightness to this easy, one-dish meal.

2 tablespoons olive oil

3 garlic cloves, minced

4 boneless, skinless chicken breasts

1 cup couscous

½ teaspoon salt

¼ teaspoon freshly ground black pepper

Juice of 3 lemons

¼ cup finely chopped flat-leaf parsley

¼ cup Quick-Pickled Onions (page 155), finely chopped

NUT-FREE
DAIRY-FREE
SOY-FREE

Active Time: 10 minutes
Total Time: 30 minutes

Yield: 4 servings
Serving size: 1¼ cups

1. In a large skillet, heat the olive oil over medium heat. Add the garlic, sautéing it for 2 minutes.

2. Add 1½ cups water to the skillet and increase the heat to high, letting the water come to a simmer.

3. Add the chicken to the water, lower the heat to medium-low, and cover the skillet. Allow the chicken to cook for 15 minutes, or until an instant-read thermometer inserted into the thickest part of the chicken reaches 165°F.

4. Use tongs to carefully transfer the chicken to a serving plate. Cover with foil to keep warm.

5. Add the couscous to the remaining water in the skillet, along with the salt, pepper, and lemon juice. Cover the skillet, turn off the heat, and let the couscous sit to absorb the water for 5 minutes.

6. Use a fork to fluff the couscous. Serve it with the cooked chicken, topped with the chopped parsley and pickled onions.

Per serving: Total calories: 334; total fat: 10g; saturated fat: 2g; carbohydrates: 37g; sugar: 1g; fiber: 2g; protein: 29g; sodium: 475mg; cholesterol: 65mg

Unbreaded Chicken Marsala

This healthier version of this dish skips the breading but not the flavor. The chicken stays tender because it's cooked in a skillet with olive oil and Marsala wine. The result is a delicious chicken dish that can be served with cooked pasta, mashed potatoes, or steamed vegetables for a satisfying meal.

4 boneless, skinless chicken breasts

½ teaspoon sea salt

¼ teaspoon freshly ground black pepper

2 tablespoons olive oil

1 onion, chopped

1 cup button mushrooms, sliced

½ teaspoon dried oregano

1½ cup Marsala wine

NUT-FREE
GLUTEN-FREE
DAIRY-FREE
SOY-FREE

Active Time: 20 minutes

Total Time: 25 minutes

Yield: 4 servings
Serving size: 1 cup

TIP: If you don't want to flatten the chicken, you'll need to add 3 minutes of cooking time to each side.

1. Use a sharp knife to cut each chicken breast in half lengthwise. Then, lay the chicken slices on a cutting board and cover them with a piece of plastic wrap. Use a mallet to pound the chicken pieces flat.
2. Season the chicken with the salt and pepper.
3. In a large skillet, heat the olive oil over medium heat.
4. Add the chicken and cook for 5 minutes on each side.
5. Transfer to a serving plate, covering it with foil to keep warm.
6. Add the onion, mushrooms, and oregano to the skillet and sauté for 3 minutes.
7. Add the wine and cook for 2 minutes.
8. Turn off the heat, add the chicken back to the skillet, and toss to coat everything with the sauce. Serve hot.

Per serving: Total calories: 248; total fat: 12g; saturated fat: 2g; carbohydrates: 5g; sugar: 3g; fiber: 1g; protein: 33g; sodium: 560mg; cholesterol: 86mg

Turkey Parmesan Meatballs

Meatballs are such a versatile food. You can serve them on top of cooked pasta or zucchini noodles, salad or mashed potatoes. These meatballs are full of Parmesan flavor.

1 pound ground turkey

½ onion, chopped

1 egg, beaten

¼ cup grated Parmesan cheese

½ teaspoon dried parsley flakes

¼ teaspoon sea salt

¼ teaspoon freshly ground black pepper

⅛ teaspoon garlic powder

NUT-FREE
GLUTEN-FREE
SOY-FREE
KIDS LOVE IT
FREEZER FRIENDLY

Active Time: 10 minutes
Total Time: 30 minutes

Yield: 12 meatballs
Serving size: 4 meatballs

1. Preheat the oven to 375°F. Line a baking sheet with parchment paper and set aside.

2. In a large mixing bowl, combine the turkey, onion, egg, Parmesan, parsley flakes, salt, pepper, and garlic powder.

3. Use your hands to mix the ingredients together, and then form 12 meatballs.

4. Lay each meatball on the baking sheet, leaving a little bit of room between each meatball. Bake them for 20 minutes.

5. Serve hot.

TIP: To freeze the cooked meatballs, let them cool completely. Put them in a zip-top bag and store in the freezer for up to 2 months. Defrost the meatballs completely in the refrigerator and reheat in the microwave before serving.

Per serving: Per 3 meatball serving: Total calories: 212; total fat: 11g; saturated fat: 4g; carbohydrates: 2g; sugar: 1g; fiber: <1g; protein: 26g; sodium: 365mg; cholesterol: 131mg

Basil-Turkey Meatloaf

Meatloaves are one of those dishes you can easily prepare ahead of time when you're not too busy and then pop in the oven when you're ready for a hearty meal. But this recipe is so fast that you can make it and cook it in 30 minutes. I like to serve this dish with sautéed or steamed vegetables and baked potatoes.

Nonstick cooking spray

1 pound ground turkey

¼ cup almond flour

2 teaspoons dried basil

1 egg, beaten

¼ cup ketchup, plus
2 tablespoons, divided

¼ teaspoon sea salt

¼ teaspoon freshly
ground black pepper

GLUTEN-FREE
DAIRY-FREE
FREEZER FRIENDLY

Active Time: 10 minutes
Total Time: 30 minutes

Yield: 4 servings
Serving size: One-quarter
of the meatloaf

TIP: Assemble and freeze the meatloaf before baking it for an extra-fast meal. Store in an airtight container in the freezer for up to 2 months. When you're ready to cook it, defrost overnight in the refrigerator and then bake according to the instructions provided here.

1. Preheat the oven to 425°F. Spray a 9-by-13-inch glass baking dish with nonstick cooking spray and set aside.

2. In a large mixing bowl, combine the ground turkey, almond flour, basil, egg, 2 tablespoons of ketchup, and the salt and pepper. Use your hands to mix until well combined.

3. Transfer the mixture to the baking dish. Use a spatula to flatten the top of the meatloaf.

4. Spoon ¼ cup of ketchup over the top of the meatloaf, spreading it evenly.

5. Bake the meatloaf for 22 minutes, or until the liquid at the bottom of the pan is bubbling. Serve it hot.

Per serving: Total calories: 250; total fat: 13g; saturated fat: 3g; carbohydrates: 10g; sugar: <1g; fiber: 1g; protein: 25g; sodium: 488mg; cholesterol: 127mg

Pineapple Turkey Burgers

This recipe always reminds me of vacationing in Hawaii, where pineapple seems to be a part of almost every meal. These burgers are moist and full of tropical flavor and may immediately transport you back to your favorite topical vacation, making them perfect for anytime you need to catch your breath and unwind.

1½ pounds ground turkey

½ onion, minced

1 egg, beaten

1 tablespoon reduced-sodium tamari

½ teaspoon ground ginger

½ teaspoon dried garlic

¼ teaspoon sea salt

¼ teaspoon ground black pepper

1 (20-ounce) can pineapple slices, drained

4 burger buns, sliced in half

NUT-FREE
DAIRY-FREE
FREEZER FRIENDLY

Active Time: 10 minutes

Total Time: 30 minutes

Yield: 6 burgers
Serving size: 1 burger

TIP: To freeze the cooked burgers, let them come to room temperature and then put them in a zip-top bag. These will keep in the freezer for up to 2 months. You can reheat the burgers in the microwave or in a skillet on the stove top.

1. Preheat the oven to 400°F. Line a baking sheet with parchment paper and set aside.

2. In a large mixing bowl, use your hands to combine the ground turkey, onion, egg, tamari, ginger, garlic, salt, and pepper. Form 6 medium patties.

3. Lay the patties on the baking sheet and bake for 20 minutes, flipping the patties once halfway through. The burgers will be a golden color when they are cooked through.

4. While the burgers are cooking, toast the bun halves in a toaster oven or on a nonstick skillet.

5. Serve the burgers hot, on the buns, with two or three pineapple slices on top of each burger.

Per serving: Total calories: 344; total fat: 13g; saturated fat: 4g; carbohydrates: 21g; sugar: 17g; fiber: 2g; protein: 35g; sodium: 479mg; cholesterol: 167mg

Honey and Garlic Turkey Sloppy Joes

Sloppy Joes are so tasty because of their sweet-and-sour flavor. This version uses ground turkey with just enough honey to deliver that authentic sweetness. It also includes grated carrot for a hidden vegetable. Serve this delicious Sloppy Joe recipe on toasted hamburger buns or on top of rice or mashed potatoes for a wheat-free option.

1 tablespoon olive oil

1 pound ground turkey

3 carrots, grated

½ onion, chopped

3 garlic cloves, minced

3 tablespoons ketchup

2 tablespoons honey

2 tablespoons reduced-sodium tamari

2 tablespoons apple cider vinegar

NUT-FREE
GLUTEN-FREE
DAIRY-FREE
KIDS LOVE IT

Active Time: 15 minutes
Total Time: 25 minutes

Yield: 4 servings
Serving size: 1 cup

1. In a large skillet, heat the olive oil over medium heat.

2. Add the turkey, carrots, onion, and garlic and sauté for 5 minutes. Use a spatula to break apart the meat as it cooks.

3. Stir in the ketchup, honey, tamari, and apple cider vinegar.

4. Turn the heat to low, cover the skillet, and let it simmer for an additional 5 minutes.

5. Serve hot.

Per serving: Total calories: 272; total fat: 12g; saturated fat: 3g; carbohydrates: 19g; sugar: 11g; fiber: 2g; protein: 24g; sodium: 588mg; cholesterol: 80mg

Loaded Chicken and Black Bean Nachos

These healthy nachos use ground chicken and just enough cheese. The black beans and green chiles add nutrition and flavor. Trust me, nobody will complain when you tell them you're serving nachos for dinner.

1 tablespoon olive oil

1 pound ground chicken

½ onion, chopped

½ teaspoon chili powder

½ teaspoon dried oregano

1 (15-ounce) can black beans, rinsed and drained

1 (4-ounce) can diced green chiles, drained

1 (16-ounce) bag corn tortilla chips

1 cup shredded Cheddar cheese

NUT-FREE
GLUTEN-FREE
SOY-FREE
KIDS LOVE IT

Active Time: 20 minutes
Total Time: 30 minutes

Yield: 5 servings
Serving size: About 10 chips

TIP: Be sure to look for corn tortilla chips that are gluten-free.

1. Preheat the oven to 375°F. Line two baking sheets with parchment paper and set aside.

2. In a large skillet, heat the olive oil over medium heat.

3. Add the chicken, onion, chili powder, and dried oregano and cook for 5 minutes, using a spatula to break apart the meat as it cooks.

4. Turn off the heat and add the black beans and green chiles, stirring to combine.

5. Spread the chips on the baking sheets. Use a slotted serving spoon to scoop the chicken-and-bean mixture onto the chips.

6. Sprinkle the cheese on top of the nachos. Bake them for 10 minutes, or until the cheese has melted.

7. Serve hot.

Per serving: Total calories: 817; total fat: 43g; saturated fat: 12g; carbohydrates: 75g; sugar: 2g; fiber: 11g; protein: 33g; sodium: 758mg; cholesterol: 96mg

Cabbage Egg Roll in a Bowl

Almost everyone loves the flavor and crunch of egg rolls, and this bowl replicates their yummy cabbage filling. The flavors go great with the chicken and veggies. This Cabbage Egg Roll in a Bowl is so much healthier than actual egg rolls, which are deep-fried—so, the next time your egg roll cravings hit, make this instead.

1 tablespoon olive oil

1 onion, chopped

1 pound ground chicken

1 (14-ounce) bag shredded cabbage

¼ cup reduced-sodium tamari

2 teaspoons Sriracha

1 teaspoon rice wine vinegar

½ teaspoon ground ginger

1 teaspoon toasted sesame oil

2 scallions, sliced

NUT-FREE
GLUTEN-FREE
DAIRY-FREE

Active Time: 15 minutes
Total Time: 25 minutes

Yield: 4 servings
Serving size: 1¼ cups

TIP: If you can't find bagged shredded cabbage, bagged coleslaw mix will work, too.

1. In a large skillet, heat the olive oil over medium heat. Add the onion and ground chicken and cook for 5 minutes, using a spatula to break up the chicken as it cooks.

2. Add the cabbage, tamari, Sriracha, vinegar, and ground ginger, stirring to combine. Cook for an additional 5 minutes, or until the cabbage is tender.

3. Turn off the heat and stir in the sesame oil. Top the dish with the sliced scallions and serve hot.

Per serving: Total calories: 279; total fat: 17g; saturated fat: 4g; carbohydrates: 7g; sugar: 3g; fiber: 2g; protein: 24g; sodium: 827mg; cholesterol: 95mg

Easy Chicken Tikka Masala

This is the dish that I order whenever I visit an Indian restaurant. It's full of rich flavor, without being too spicy. Served with a nice flatbread or steamed basmati rice, this is my idea of easy dinner perfection, and it makes for great leftovers, too.

2 tablespoons olive oil

4 boneless, skinless chicken breasts, cut into 1-inch chunks

1 onion, diced

3 garlic cloves, minced

1 tablespoon garam masala

½ teaspoon ground ginger

1 (14.5-ounce) can tomato sauce

1 cup reduced-sodium chicken broth

½ cup heavy cream (for dairy-free option, use coconut milk)

2 tablespoons chopped fresh cilantro, for topping

NUT-FREE
GLUTEN-FREE
DAIRY-FREE
SOY-FREE

Active Time: 15 minutes
Total Time: 25 minutes

Yield: 4 servings
Serving size: 1 cup

TIP: If you don't have garam masala, you can use 1 tablespoon of ground curry instead.

1. In a large skillet, heat the olive oil over medium heat.
2. Add the chicken, onion, garlic, garam masala, and ground ginger and sauté for 5 minutes, stirring often.
3. Add the tomato sauce and chicken broth, stirring to combine the ingredients. Turn the heat to low, cover the skillet, and allow everything to cook for an additional 8 minutes.
4. Turn off the heat and stir in the heavy cream.
5. Serve hot, with the cilantro sprinkled on top.

Per serving: Total calories: 332; total fat: 21g; saturated fat: 8g; carbohydrates: 12g; sugar: 6g; fiber: 2g; protein: 25g; sodium: 1,050mg; cholesterol: 106mg

Orange Chicken Stir-Fry

This recipe is perfectly suited for busy days when you are really short on time. You can use whatever blend of frozen stir-fry vegetables you prefer. I like ones that include broccoli, bell pepper, and mushrooms. Serve this dish plain or over steamed rice.

4 tablespoons olive oil, divided

4 boneless, skinless chicken breasts, cut into bite-size pieces

1 (16-ounce) bag frozen stir-fry vegetables

Juice of 2 oranges (about ½ cup)

2 tablespoons reduced-sodium tamari

2 tablespoons rice vinegar

1 tablespoon brown sugar

¼ teaspoon ground ginger

¼ teaspoon garlic powder

¼ cup cashews, chopped

GLUTEN-FREE
DAIRY-FREE
KIDS LOVE IT

Active Time: 10 minutes
Total Time: 25 minutes

Yield: **4 servings**
Serving size: **1½ cups**

TIP: Look for bags of frozen stir-fry vegetables in the frozen section of your grocery store.

1. In a large skillet, heat 2 tablespoons of oil in a large skillet over medium heat. Add the chicken pieces and cook for 5 minutes, stirring occasionally so the chicken cooks evenly on all sides.

2. Use a slotted spoon to transfer the chicken to a plate, then heat the remaining 2 tablespoons of olive oil in the same skillet.

3. Add the frozen vegetables and cook for 7 minutes, stirring occasionally.

4. In a medium mixing bowl, whisk together the orange juice, tamari, vinegar, brown sugar, ground ginger, and garlic powder.

5. Transfer the chicken back into the skillet and pour the orange juice sauce over the mixture.

6. Put a lid on the skillet and cook for another 2 minutes to warm the sauce.

7. Turn off the heat and sprinkle the cashews over the top. Serve hot.

Per serving: Total calories: 335; total fat: 21g; saturated fat: 3g; carbohydrates: 14g; sugar: 7g; fiber: 2g; protein: 27g; sodium: 601mg; cholesterol: 65mg

Chicken Satay and Veggie Stir-Fry

A stir-fry is a great way to get a healthy dinner on the table that includes lots of vegetables. The creamy peanut satay sauce is super easy to make and brings all the flavors of the chicken and the veggies together. Your kids might even surprise you by asking for seconds of this delicious chicken recipe.

4 tablespoons olive oil, divided

4 boneless, skinless chicken breasts, cut into bite-size pieces

1 onion, chopped

1 red bell pepper, sliced

1 carrot, julienned

2 cups sugar snap peas

3 garlic cloves, minced

⅓ cup peanut butter

2 tablespoons reduced-sodium tamari

2 tablespoons rice vinegar

2 tablespoons brown sugar

GLUTEN-FREE
DAIRY-FREE
KIDS LOVE IT

Active Time: 20 minutes
Total Time: 30 minutes

Yield: **4 servings**
Serving size: **1½ cups**

TIP: Feel free to use whatever fresh vegetables you have on hand for this dish. You will need a total of about 3½ cups of vegetables.

1. In a large skillet, heat 2 tablespoons of oil in a large skillet over medium heat. Add the chicken pieces and cook for 5 minutes, stirring occasionally so the chicken cooks evenly on all sides.

2. Use a slotted spoon to transfer the chicken to a plate. Then, heat the remaining 2 tablespoons of olive oil in the same skillet.

3. Add the onion, bell pepper, carrot, sugar snap peas, and garlic and cook the vegetables for 5 minutes, stirring occasionally.

4. Make the peanut satay sauce while your vegetables cook by whisking together the peanut butter, tamari, rice vinegar, and brown sugar in a small mixing bowl until fully combined.

5. Put the chicken back into the skillet and pour the peanut satay sauce over the mixture.

6. Put a lid on the skillet and cook for another 5 minutes.

7. Serve hot.

Per serving: Total calories: 438; total fat: 27g; saturated fat: 5g; carbohydrates: 23g; sugar: 12g; fiber: 4g; protein: 32g; sodium: 642mg; cholesterol: 65mg

Turkey Taco Pasta Skillet

This pasta dish has all the flavors of your favorite street tacos, but made into a one-pot meal. The turkey, beans, salsa, and cheese melt together with the tender pasta to create a truly comforting meal without any of the guilt.

2 tablespoons olive oil

1 onion, chopped

1 red bell pepper, chopped

3 garlic cloves, minced

1 pound ground turkey

1 teaspoon ground cumin

1 teaspoon chili powder

¼ teaspoon sea salt

¼ teaspoon freshly ground black pepper

1 (15-ounce) can pinto beans, rinsed and drained

1 cup salsa

1½ cups uncooked penne pasta (for gluten-free option, use gluten-free pasta)

1 cup shredded Cheddar cheese (omit for dairy-free option)

NUT-FREE
GLUTEN-FREE
DAIRY-FREE
SOY-FREE

Active Time: 15 minutes
Total Time: 25 minutes

Yield: 4 servings
Serving size: 1¼ cups

TIP: Leave out the chili powder if you don't like spicy foods. It will still have a lot of great flavor even without it.

1. In a large pot, heat the olive oil over medium heat. Add the onion, bell pepper, garlic, turkey, cumin, chili powder, salt, and black pepper and sauté for 5 minutes, using a spatula to break up the turkey as it cooks.

2. Add the pinto beans, 1¾ cups water, the salsa, and pasta to the pot. Turn the heat to high and let the pot come to a boil. Then turn the heat to low, cover the pot with a lid, and let the mixture cook for 8 minutes, or until the pasta has absorbed most of the liquid.

3. Turn off the heat and sprinkle the cheese over the top of the mixture. Serve hot.

Per serving: Total calories: 583; total fat: 25g; saturated fat: 10g; carbohydrates: 51g; sugar: 6g; fiber: 8g; protein: 40g; sodium: 701mg; cholesterol: 105mg

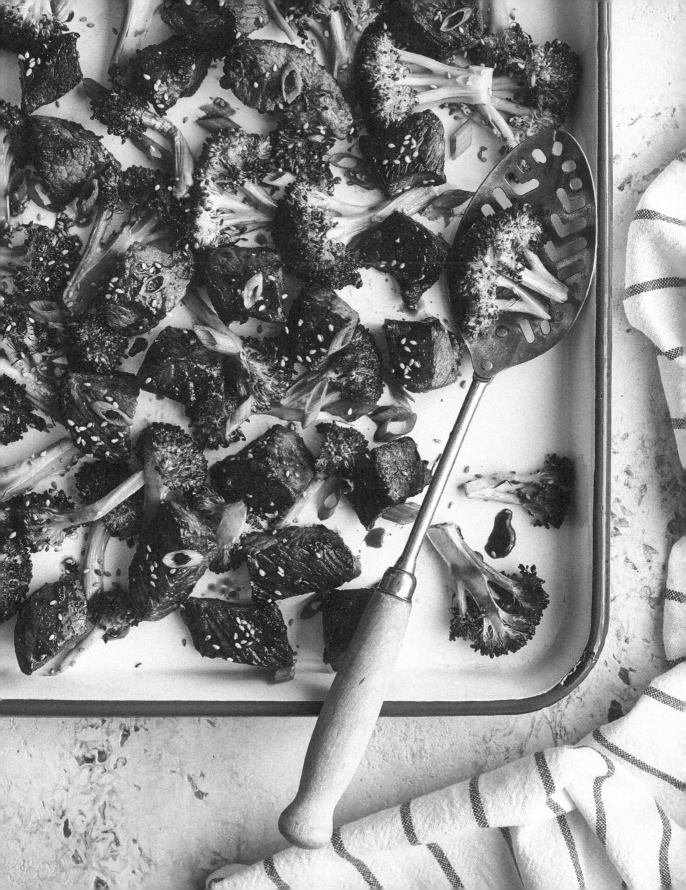

Meat

Sheet Pan Beef and Broccoli

Sausage and Cabbage Low-Carb Bowl

A few summers ago, my husband and I went on a riverboat trip through the German countryside. One of our favorite meals was from a medieval village restaurant, where we had sausages and cabbage while looking onto a thirteenth-century cathedral. It was a magical experience, and this dish reminds me of that trip.

12 ounces cooked bratwurst pork sausage (about 4 pieces), sliced

1 tablespoon olive oil

1 onion, chopped

1 medium green cabbage, thinly sliced

1 teaspoon prepared horseradish

NUT-FREE
GLUTEN-FREE
DAIRY-FREE
SOY-FREE
EXTRA QUICK

Active Time: 15 minutes
Total Time: 20 minutes

Yield: 4 servings
Serving size: One-quarter of dish

TIP: You can find cooked bratwurst sausages in the refrigerated deli section of most grocery stores. Niman Ranch makes a good one that is gluten-free.

1. In a large skillet over medium heat, sauté the sausage for 5 minutes. Use a spatula to stir the sausage occasionally to keep it from burning.

2. Transfer the sausage to a serving plate and cover with aluminum foil to keep warm.

3. Use the same skillet to heat the olive oil over medium heat. Add the onion and sauté for 2 minutes, stirring it often.

4. Add ½ cup water and the cabbage and cook for an additional 5 minutes, or until the cabbage has wilted.

5. Turn off the heat and add the sausage back into the skillet. Stir to combine.

6. Serve hot, with horseradish on the side.

Per serving: Total calories: 338; total fat: 23g; saturated fat: 8g; carbohydrates: 17g; sugar: 10g; fiber: 6g; protein: 18g; sodium: 576mg; cholesterol: 55mg

Panfried Honey Mustard Pork Chops

These versatile pork chops can be served for a casual weeknight meal or a formal dinner party. Serve them with a simple side salad or your favorite steamed vegetable. The honey mustard sauce pairs perfectly with these tender pork chops.

2 tablespoons olive oil

4 pork chops

½ teaspoon sea salt

¼ teaspoon freshly ground black pepper

2 tablespoons Dijon mustard

¼ cup honey

NUT-FREE
GLUTEN-FREE
DAIRY-FREE
SOY-FREE

Active Time: 10 minutes
Total Time: 25 minutes

Yield: 4 servings
Serving size: 1 pork chop

1. In a large skillet, heat the olive oil over medium heat.
2. Add the pork chops, season them with the salt and pepper, and sauté for 5 minutes. Put a lid on the skillet while the pork chops cook.
3. In a small mixing bowl, whisk together the mustard and the honey.
4. Turn the pork chops over and spoon the honey mustard sauce over the top of the chops.
5. Put the lid back on the skillet, reduce the heat to low, and cook them for an additional 10 minutes.
6. Serve hot.

Per serving: Total calories: 272; total fat: 13g; saturated fat: 4g; carbohydrates: 18g; sugar: 17g; fiber: 1g; protein: 21g; sodium: 722mg; cholesterol: 45mg

Pork and Stir-Fry Vegetable Bowl

If you're like me, sometimes you run out of fresh vegetables and need to raid the freezer. This recipe uses frozen stir-fry vegetables combined with cooked pork and a sweet-and-sour sauce. It's an easy way to get a healthy dinner on the table.

1 tablespoon olive oil

1 (12-ounce) bag frozen stir-fry vegetables

1 pound ground pork

2 tablespoons reduced-sodium tamari

1 tablespoon hoisin sauce

1 tablespoon toasted sesame oil

NUT-FREE
DAIRY-FREE
EXTRA QUICK

Active Time: 15 minutes
Total Time: 20 minutes

Yield: 4 servings
Serving size: 1 pork chop

TIP: You can find frozen bags of stir-fry vegetables in the frozen aisle of your grocery store.

1. In a large skillet, heat the olive oil over medium heat. Add the frozen vegetables and cook for 7 minutes, or until the vegetables are tender. Transfer to a serving bowl and cover with foil to keep warm.

2. Add the pork to the skillet. Cook for 6 minutes, using a spatula to break up the meat as it cooks.

3. Turn off the heat and stir in the tamari, hoisin sauce, and toasted sesame oil.

4. Serve hot.

Per serving: Total calories: 393; total fat: 31g; saturated fat: 10g; carbohydrates: 5g; sugar: 3g; fiber: 2g; protein: 21g; sodium: 489mg; cholesterol: 82mg

Beef Burgers with Portobello Buns

This recipe uses portobello mushroom caps instead of a hamburger bun to serve thick and juicy beef burgers. I recommend eating these burgers with a fork and a knife, as opposed to picking them up and taking a bite as you would a traditional burger. However you decide to eat them, I think you're going to love this healthy twist on burgers.

4 portobello mushrooms, wiped clean with a dry paper towel

Nonstick cooking spray

1 pound lean ground beef

1 egg, beaten

1 teaspoon Dijon mustard

½ teaspoon garlic powder

½ teaspoon sea salt

¼ teaspoon freshly ground black pepper

NUT-FREE
GLUTEN-FREE
DAIRY-FREE
SOY-FREE

Active Time: 20 minutes
Total Time: 25 minutes

1. Preheat the oven to 425°F. Line a baking sheet with parchment paper and set aside.

2. Use a spoon to carefully remove the gills from the mushrooms. Lay the mushrooms, cap-side up on the baking sheet. Lightly spray the mushrooms caps with nonstick cooking spray.

3. Bake the mushrooms for 10 minutes, or until they start to brown on all sides.

4. Make the burgers while the mushrooms bake by combining the ground beef, eggs, mustard, garlic powder, salt, and pepper in a medium mixing bowl. Use your hands to form 4 burger patties.

5. Heat a large nonstick skillet over medium heat. Add the burger patties and cook them for 4 minutes on each side. Put a lid on the skillet to prevent any grease from splattering.

6. Serve the burgers on top of the mushrooms.

Yield: 4 servings
Serving size: 1 burger

TIP: If you have access to a grill, you can cook both the mushrooms and the burgers on it. The mushrooms will only need to cook for about 3 minutes to create grill marks, and the burgers will need about 3 minutes per side.

Per serving: Total calories: 233; total fat: 11g; saturated fat: 4g; carbohydrates: 5g; sugar: 2g; fiber: 1g; protein: 27g; sodium: 414mg; cholesterol: 117mg

Barbecue Meatloaf Muffins

A typical meatloaf can take up to an hour to cook in the oven. I've cut the baking time way down by making the meatloaf in a muffin tin. What you get are individual portions of your favorite classic dish. Kids love these savory meatloaf muffins, too.

Nonstick cooking spray

1 pound lean ground beef

½ onion, minced

2 garlic cloves, minced

1 egg, beaten

⅓ cup almond flour

¼ cup prepared barbecue sauce or Easy Homemade Barbecue Sauce (page 156)

¼ teaspoon sea salt

¼ teaspoon freshly ground black pepper

GLUTEN-FREE
DAIRY-FREE
SOY-FREE
KIDS LOVE IT
FREEZER FRIENDLY

Active Time: 15 minutes
Total Time: 25 minutes

1. Preheat the oven to 375°F. Spray a 12-cup muffin tin with nonstick cooking spray and set aside.

2. In a medium mixing bowl, combine the ground beef, onion, garlic, egg, almond flour, barbecue sauce, salt, and pepper. Use your hands to combine the ingredients.

3. Divide the meatloaf mixture between the 12 muffin wells. Bake them for 20 minutes, or until the muffins are cooked through. Serve this dish hot.

Yield: 4 servings
Serving size: 3 muffins

TIP: To freeze the muffins, let them cool completely, and then put them in a zip-top bag. Store in the freezer for up to 2 months.

Per serving: Total calories: 280; total fat: 16g; saturated fat: 5g; carbohydrates: 6g; sugar: 6g; fiber: 2g; protein: 27g; sodium: 361mg; cholesterol: 117mg

Basil Beef with Cauliflower Rice

This lower-carb, extra-quick dish uses cauliflower rice instead of regular steamed rice. Cauliflower rice has a fairly neutral flavor and a similar texture to rice. This is one of my favorite meals to prep. I make a double batch and then pack up the leftovers in reheatable containers to enjoy for several days.

2 tablespoons olive oil

1 (14-ounce) bag cauliflower rice

1 pound lean ground beef

1 onion, chopped

3 garlic cloves, minced

2 tablespoons reduced-sodium tamari

2 tablespoons rice vinegar

¼ cup chopped basil leaves (from about 15 leaves)

¼ teaspoon red pepper flakes

¼ teaspoon ground ginger

NUT-FREE
GLUTEN-FREE
DAIRY-FREE
EXTRA QUICK

Active Time: 10 minutes
Total Time: 20 minutes

Yield: **4 servings**
Serving size: 1½ cups

TIP: If you can't find fresh bagged cauliflower rice, you can use frozen cauliflower rice and prepare it in the microwave according to the directions on the package.

1. In a large skillet, heat the olive oil over medium heat. Add the cauliflower rice, cover the skillet with a lid, and cook for about 5 minutes.

2. Transfer the cooked cauliflower rice to a serving bowl and cover with aluminum foil to keep warm.

3. Heat the skillet over medium heat and add the ground beef, onion, and garlic. Cook them for 6 minutes, using a spatula to break apart the meat as it cooks.

4. Reduce the heat to low and add the tamari, rice vinegar, basil, red pepper flakes, and ground ginger. Stir to combine.

5. Pour the cooked cauliflower back into the skillet with the beef mixture and cook for an additional 2 minutes.

6. Serve hot.

Per serving: Total calories: 289; total fat: 17g; saturated fat: 5g; carbohydrates: 6g; sugar: 2g; fiber: 2g; protein: 27g; sodium: 589mg; cholesterol: 70mg

Sheet Pan Beef and Broccoli

This quick and easy Asian-inspired dish is made using the sheet pan method. The ingredients get coated with the sweet and spicy homemade sauce, and then baked until the meat is cooked through and the veggies are still crisp. I like to serve this dish over cooked white or brown rice.

1 pound sirloin steak, cut into 1-inch chunks

4 cups broccoli florets

¼ cup reduced-sodium tamari

1 tablespoon olive oil

1 tablespoon brown sugar

1 tablespoon rice vinegar

½ teaspoon garlic powder

½ teaspoon red pepper flakes

3 scallions, chopped

1 tablespoon toasted sesame seeds

NUT-FREE
GLUTEN-FREE
DAIRY-FREE

Active Time: 10 minutes
Total Time: 25 minutes

Yield: 4 servings
Serving size: 1¼ cups

TIP: To toast the sesame seeds, heat a small non-stick skillet over low heat. Add the sesame seeds and let them toast for about 2 minutes, being careful to not let them burn.

1. Preheat the oven to 425°F. Line a baking sheet with aluminum foil and set aside.

2. In a large mixing bowl, combine the steak, broccoli, tamari, olive oil, brown sugar, rice vinegar, garlic powder, and red pepper flakes. Stir to combine, making sure that all the beef and broccoli get coated with the sauce.

3. Put the beef and broccoli onto the sheet pan. Use a spoon to spread the ingredients into a flat layer. Bake the mixture for 15 minutes, or until the meat has cooked through and the vegetables have started to brown.

4. Remove the baking sheet from the oven and top the mixture with the scallions and toasted sesame seeds. Serve hot.

Per serving: Total calories: 340; total fat: 21g; saturated fat: 7g; carbohydrates: 10g; sugar: 4g; fiber: 3g; protein: 26g; sodium: 781mg; cholesterol: 76mg

One-Dish Pepper Steak Skillet

This one-dish meal combines tender steak pieces with flavorful and colorful sliced bell peppers. Crunchy onion and a homemade honey mustard sauce brings the flavors all together. Serve this dish on its own or with my Golden Rice Pilaf (page 157).

1 pound sirloin steak, thinly sliced

1 tablespoon olive oil

1 onion, chopped

3 garlic cloves, minced

1 red bell pepper, sliced

1 green bell pepper, sliced

2 tablespoons apple cider vinegar

1 tablespoon Dijon mustard

2 tablespoons honey

½ teaspoon sea salt

¼ teaspoon freshly ground black pepper

NUT-FREE
GLUTEN-FREE
DAIRY-FREE
SOY-FREE
EXTRA QUICK

Active Time: 20 minutes
Total Time: 25 minutes

Yield: 4 servings
Serving size: 1¼ cups

TIP: You can use whatever combination of red, green, orange, or yellow bell peppers you prefer for this recipe.

1. In a large, nonstick skillet over heat, cook the steak for 5 minutes, stirring occasionally so it cooks on all sides.

2. Transfer the steak to a serving plate and cover with foil to keep warm.

3. Pour the olive oil into the skillet and heat over medium heat. Add the onion, garlic, red bell pepper, and green bell pepper and stir to combine. Sauté for 3 minutes, or until the vegetables start to soften.

4. Turn the heat to low and add the vinegar, mustard, honey, salt, and pepper. Stir to combine.

5. Return the cooked steak to the skillet and toss with the vegetables and sauce.

6. Serve hot.

Per serving: Total calories: 336; total fat: 21g; saturated fat: 7g; carbohydrates: 16g; sugar: 11g; fiber: 2g; protein: 23g; sodium: 444mg; cholesterol: 76mg

Skillet Lasagna

When you're short on time but looking for a delicious dish with hidden vegetables, give this recipe a whirl. Carrots and zucchini are cooked on the stove top in a delicious meat sauce with tender lasagna noodles and topped with cheese. Serve it with a simple green salad on the side, and nobody will guess that you made this in 30 minutes.

1 tablespoon olive oil

2 carrots, shredded

1 zucchini, shredded

½ onion, finely diced

3 garlic cloves, minced

1 pound lean ground beef

½ teaspoon dried oregano

1 (14-ounce) can crushed tomatoes, with juices

8 ounces lasagna noodles (about 8 noodles), broken in half

1 cup shredded mozzarella cheese

NUT-FREE
SOY-FREE
KIDS LOVE IT

Active Time: 15 minutes
Total Time: 30 minutes

Yield: 4 servings
Serving size: One-quarter of dish

TIP: If you don't have a food processor, you can use a large cheese grater to shred the carrot and zucchini.

1. In a large skillet, heat the oil over medium heat. Add the carrots, zucchini, onion, and garlic and sauté for 3 minutes.

2. Add the ground meat and oregano and cook for an additional 5 minutes, using a spatula to break up the meat as it cooks.

3. Add the tomatoes, 3 cups of water, and the lasagna noodles and stir gently to combine.

4. Bring to a simmer, turn the heat to low, and cover the skillet. Cook for an additional 15 minutes, or until the noodle are cooked through.

5. Turn off the heat and sprinkle the cheese on top. Serve hot.

Per serving: Total calories: 557; total fat: 20g; saturated fat: 8g; carbohydrates: 53g; sugar: 7g; fiber: 5g; protein: 42g; sodium: 418mg; cholesterol: 85mg

Taco Salad Beef Skillet

This dish is a healthier version of the taco salads that are often served in fried tortilla bowls. This recipe leaves out the fried ingredients but keeps all the great flavors of a taco salad. You can always serve this dish with a side of baked tortilla chips for even more authentic flavor.

1 tablespoon olive oil

1 pound lean ground beef

1 onion, chopped

1 jalapeño pepper, seeded and finely chopped

2 garlic cloves, minced

1 teaspoon ground cumin

½ teaspoon sea salt

¼ teaspoon freshly ground black pepper

1 (15-ounce) canned pinto beans, rinsed and drained

1 cup shredded Cheddar cheese (leave out for dairy-free option)

2 cups shredded romaine lettuce

1 cup prepared or homemade Pico de Gallo (page 149)

NUT-FREE
GLUTEN-FREE
DAIRY-FREE
SOY-FREE
KIDS LOVE IT

Active Time: 16 minutes
Total Time: 23 minutes

Yield: 4 servings
Serving size: 1½ cups

TIP: Leave out the jalapeño pepper if you don't like spicy foods.

1. In a large skillet, heat the olive oil over medium heat.

2. Add the beef, onion, jalapeño, garlic, cumin, salt, and pepper and sauté for 6 minutes. Use a spatula to break up the meat as it cooks.

3. Mix in the pinto beans, stirring to combine. Turn the heat to low, cover the skillet, and cook for an additional 5 minutes.

4. Turn off the heat and sprinkle the cheese and romaine over the mixture. Serve hot with pico de gallo.

Per serving: Total calories: 461; total fat: 23g; saturated fat: 11g; carbohydrates: 26g; sugar: 4g; fiber: 7g; protein: 37g; sodium: 700mg; cholesterol: 95mg

Mediterranean Beef Bowl

If you've ever had Greek-style kebabs, then you'll love this dish, which captures all those flavors. The spices add warmth, and the chickpeas help round out the flavor and nutritional profiles. Serve it with a creamy yogurt tzatziki sauce, and you'll swear you've landed on a Greek island.

1 tablespoon olive oil

½ onion, chopped

3 garlic cloves, minced

1 pound lean ground beef

1 teaspoon ground cumin

½ teaspoon sea salt

¼ teaspoon freshly ground black pepper

¼ teaspoon red pepper flakes

¼ teaspoon ground cinnamon

1 (15-ounce) can chickpeas rinsed and drained

¼ cup chopped fresh flat-leaf parsley

1 cup Tzatziki Yogurt Sauce (page 150) (leave out for dairy-free option)

NUT-FREE
GLUTEN-FREE
DAIRY-FREE
SOY-FREE

Active Time: 12 minutes
Total Time: 22 minutes

Yield: 4 servings
Serving size: 1¼ cups

TIP: For extra nutrition and texture, I like to serve the beef on top of crispy, chopped romaine lettuce. You can also serve it on top of white or brown rice, pasta, or sautéed cauliflower rice.

1. In a large skillet, heat the oil over medium heat. Add the onion and garlic and sauté for 3 minutes, stirring occasionally.

2. Add the beef, cumin, salt, pepper, red pepper flakes, and cinnamon and cook for an additional 7 minutes. Use a spatula to break up the meat as it cooks.

3. Turn the heat to low and add the chickpeas. Stir to combine. Cover the skillet and cook for 3 minutes more, until the beans are warmed through.

4. Turn off the heat and top the dish with the fresh, chopped parsley. Serve hot with the tzatziki on the side.

Per serving: Total calories: 374; total fat: 17g; saturated fat: 6g; carbohydrates: 25g; sugar: 6g; fiber: 6g; protein: 31g; sodium: 457mg; cholesterol: 75mg

Spaghetti with Quick Bolognese

At the end of the week, when my kitchen supplies are running low, I turn to this easy spaghetti dish that doesn't require a lot of fresh ingredients. The meat sauce is made with ground beef and crushed tomatoes with onion, garlic, and oregano added for flavoring. Everyone who tries it loves this classic, hearty dish.

1 (8-ounce) package spaghetti (for gluten-free option, use gluten-free spaghetti)

1 tablespoon olive oil

1 pound lean ground beef

3 carrots, grated

1 onion, chopped

3 garlic cloves, minced

½ teaspoon ground oregano

¼ teaspoon sea salt

¼ teaspoon freshly ground black pepper

1 (28-ounce) can crushed tomatoes, with juices

2 tablespoons tomato paste

4 tablespoons grated Parmesan cheese (omit for dairy-free option)

NUT-FREE
GLUTEN-FREE
DAIRY-FREE
SOY-FREE
KIDS LOVE IT

Active Time: 15 minutes
Total Time: 25 minutes

Yield: 4 servings
Serving size: 1½ cups

1. In a large pot, bring 8 cups of water to a boil. Add the pasta, lower the heat, and cover the pot.

2. Cook the pasta for 10 minutes, to al dente. When the pasta has finished cooking, drain it in a large colander.

3. In a large skillet, heat the oil over medium heat while the pasta cooks.

4. Add the beef, carrots, onion, garlic, oregano, salt, and pepper. Cook for 6 minutes, using a spatula to break apart the meat as it cooks.

5. Add the crushed tomatoes and tomato paste to the pot and stir to combine. Bring to a simmer, lower the heat, cover, and cook for another 5 minutes.

6. Turn off the heat. Pour the cooked pasta into the skillet and toss to combine.

7. Serve hot, with a tablespoon of grated Parmesan on top of each serving.

Per serving: Total calories: 565; total fat: 17g; saturated fat: 6g; carbohydrates: 65g; sugar: 12g; fiber: 7g; protein: 37g; sodium: 742mg; cholesterol: 75mg

Beef and Spinach Pasta Skillet

This delicious skillet meal checks all the boxes of being healthy, easy, and satisfying. The pasta gets cooked separately and then added to the simple meat sauce, which also includes chopped spinach. I like to serve this Italian-style meal with a simple green salad.

1 (16-ounce) package rotini pasta (for gluten-free option, use gluten-free pasta)

1 tablespoon olive oil

½ onion, chopped

3 garlic cloves, minced

1 pound lean ground beef

3 cups baby spinach, chopped

1 (14-ounce) can diced tomatoes, with juices

½ teaspoon ground oregano

½ teaspoon red pepper flakes

½ teaspoon sea salt

¼ teaspoon freshly ground black pepper

¼ cup grated Parmesan cheese

NUT-FREE
GLUTEN-FREE
SOY-FREE

Active Time: 15 minutes
Total Time: 25 minutes

Yield: 4 servings
Serving size: 1½ cups

TIP: You can use whatever type of pasta you prefer, including shells, elbows, or farfalle.

1. In a large pot, bring 8 cups of water to a boil. Add the pasta, lower the heat, and cover the pot.

2. Cook the pasta for 10 minutes, to al dente. When the pasta has finished cooking, drain it in a large colander.

3. While the pasta cooks, heat the oil over medium heat in a large skillet. Add the onion and garlic and sauté for 2 minutes.

4. Add the beef and cook for 7 minutes, using a spatula to break up the meat as it cooks.

5. Turn the heat to low and add the spinach, diced tomatoes, oregano, red pepper flakes, salt, and pepper.

6. Put the lid on the skillet and cook for an additional 5 minutes, or until the sauce is simmering and the spinach has completely wilted.

7. Turn off the heat, pour the cooked pasta into the skillet, and sprinkle on the Parmesan cheese. Serve hot.

Per serving: Total calories: 710; total fat: 17g; saturated fat: 6g; carbohydrates: 94g; sugar: 8g; fiber: 5g; protein: 42g; sodium: 775mg; cholesterol: 75mg

Teriyaki Beef and Noodle Bowls

This dish reminds me of my favorite take-out restaurant during college. This version is healthier, using fresh vegetables and less salt and sugar than you would find in similar restaurant dishes. The result is simply delicious and very satisfying.

1 (8-ounce) package spaghetti (for gluten-free option, use gluten-free spaghetti)

1 tablespoon olive oil

1 pound beef sirloin steak, cut into thin strips (visible fat removed)

1 onion, chopped

2 cups broccoli florets

3 garlic cloves, minced

⅓ cup reduced-sodium tamari

2 tablespoons rice wine vinegar

2 tablespoons coconut sugar

1 tablespoon cornstarch

¼ teaspoon ground ginger

NUT-FREE
GLUTEN-FREE
DAIRY-FREE

Active Time: 15 minutes
Total Time: 25 minutes

Yield: 4 servings
Serving size: 1½ cups

TIP: You can use whatever fresh vegetables you prefer, but you will need a total of about 3 cups of vegetables.

1. In a large pot, bring 8 cups of water to a boil. Add the pasta, lower the heat, and cover the pot.

2. Cook the pasta for 10 minutes, to al dente. When the pasta has finished cooking, drain it in a large colander.

3. While the pasta cooks, heat the oil over medium heat in a large skillet.

4. Add the beef, onion, broccoli, and garlic. Sauté for 8 minutes, or until the beef has fully cooked.

5. While the beef and vegetables are cooking, in a small bowl whisk together the tamari, vinegar, coconut sugar, cornstarch, ground ginger, and 1 tablespoon of water.

6. Turn the heat to low, stir in the sauce, and let simmer for 2 minutes more.

7. Turn off the heat, add the pasta noodles to the skillet, and stir to combine. Serve hot.

Per serving: Total calories: 527; total fat: 11g; saturated fat: 3g; carbohydrates: 57g; sugar: 10g; fiber: 3g; protein: 46g; sodium: 962mg; cholesterol: 64mg

Spicy Pork Lettuce Cups

This Asian-inspired dish uses lettuce to wrap up the spicy and tangy cooked pork. The water chestnuts add crunch and are so satisfying. Kids like these because the lettuce cups are fun to eat and the filling is not too spicy.

1 tablespoon olive oil

1 onion, chopped

1 pound ground pork

1 (8-ounce) can sliced water chestnuts, drained

2 tablespoons reduced-sodium tamari

2 tablespoons rice wine vinegar

2 tablespoons hoisin sauce

1 teaspoon Sriracha

¼ teaspoon ground ginger

3 scallions, sliced

2 tablespoons peanuts, chopped

9 large butter lettuce leaves

GLUTEN-FREE
DAIRY-FREE
KIDS LOVE IT

Active Time: 10 minutes
Total Time: 25 minutes

Yield: 3 servings
Serving size:
3 lettuce wraps

TIP: Leave out the Sriracha if you don't like spicy foods.

1. In a large skillet, heat the olive oil over medium heat. Add the onion and pork and cook for 8 minutes. Use a spatula to break apart the meat as it cooks.

2. Add the water chestnuts, tamari, vinegar, hoisin sauce, Sriracha, and ginger and stir to combine.

3. Turn the heat to low, cover the skillet, and continue to cook for an additional 5 minutes.

4. Turn off the heat and transfer the pork to a large serving bowl. Top the pork mixture with the sliced scallions and peanuts.

5. Serve the pork mixture in a serving bowl with the leaves on the side, spooning about 2 or 3 table-spoons of the cooked pork into the middle of a lettuce leaf for a serving.

Per serving: Total calories: 561; total fat: 40g; saturated fat: 13g; carbohydrates: 17g; sugar: 8g; fiber: 6g; protein: 32g; sodium: 776mg; cholesterol: 109mg

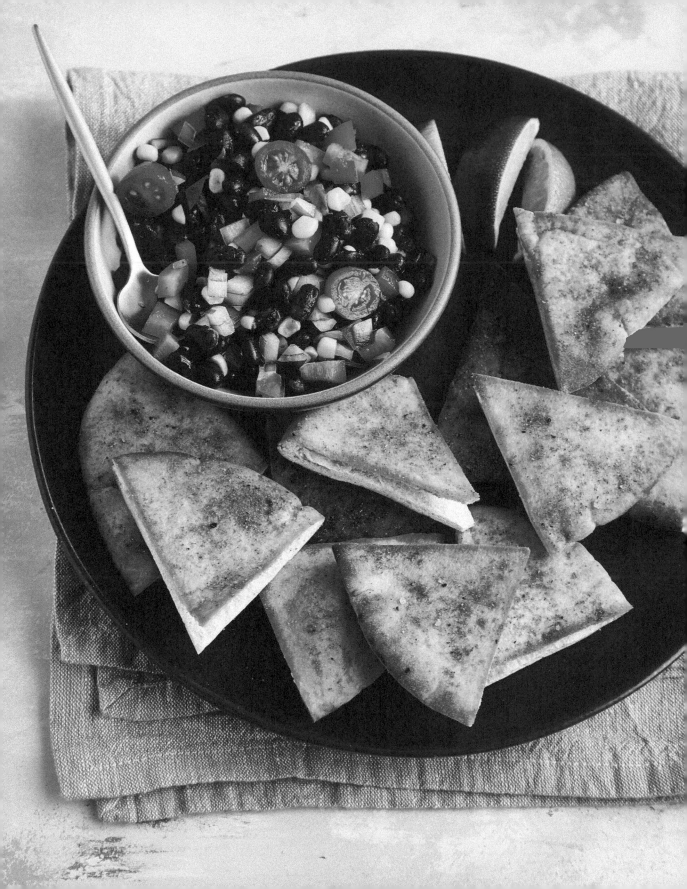

CHAPTER EIGHT

Snacks & Sides

Black Bean and Corn Salad and **Paprika Pita Chips**

Bacon-Wrapped Asparagus

Fresh asparagus stalks get a major flavor upgrade when they're wrapped in bacon. I've made this recipe healthier by wrapping the bacon around three asparagus stalks instead of just one. This low-carb side dish will go fast with any bacon lovers. This is also a great dish to serve at a party.

1 pound asparagus stalks (about 30 thin stalks), ends trimmed

½ pound bacon (regular cut), about 10 pieces

NUT-FREE
GLUTEN-FREE
DAIRY-FREE
SOY-FREE

Active Time: 12 minutes
Total Time: 22 minutes

Yield: 5 servings
Serving size: 2 bunches

1. Preheat the oven to 400°F. Line a baking sheet with parchment paper and set aside.

2. Stack 3 asparagus stalks into a bunch. Wrap 1 piece of the bacon tightly around the stalks, starting at the top and wrapping toward the bottom in a spiral. Lay the bacon-wrapped bunch on the baking sheet.

3. Repeat the previous step until all the asparagus and bacon are used up.

4. Bake the bacon-wrapped asparagus for 18 minutes, or until the bacon is fully cooked.

5. Let the asparagus and bacon cool slightly before serving.

TIP: Look for bacon brands that are preserved without nitrates. Peder-son's Natural Farms is a good brand.

Per serving: Total calories: 108; total fat: 6g; saturated fat: 2g; carbohydrates: 4g; sugar: 2g; fiber: 2g; protein: 9g; sodium: 327mg; cholesterol: 20mg

Easy Baked Kale Chips

Homemade kale chips are a crispy and salty snack that are so much healthier than fried potato chips. Kale is a superfood that is chock-full of nutrition, and baking the kale leaves transforms them into a delicious, crunchy delight. Don't be surprised if you eat the entire batch in one sitting.

1 large bunch green curly kale

2 tablespoons coconut oil, melted

½ teaspoon sea salt

NUT-FREE
GLUTEN-FREE
DAIRY-FREE
SOY-FREE
VEGAN

Active Time: 10 minutes
Total Time: 23 minutes

Yield: **4 servings**
Serving size: **1½ cups**

TIP: If you have any leftovers, let them come to room temperature before placing them in a zip-top bag and storing up to 2 days in the refrigerator.

1. Preheat the oven to 350°F. Line two baking sheets with parchment paper or aluminum foil and set aside.
2. Use your hands to tear the kale leaves from the stems. Add the leaves to a salad spinner and wash them thoroughly, then spin them dry.
3. Pat the kale dry using paper towels or a clean dish towel. Put them in a bowl and pour the coconut oil over them.
4. Use your hands to coat the kale with the oil.
5. Place the kale leaves on the baking sheets, keeping the leaves from overlapping. Sprinkle lightly with the salt.
6. Bake for 8 minutes. Flip the kale chips and return them to the oven. Let them bake for approximately 5 minutes more, or until the leaves start to become brown around the edges. Be careful not to burn them.
7. Remove the chips from the oven and serve immediately.

Per serving: Total calories: 135; total fat: 7g; saturated fat: 7g; carbohydrates: 14g; sugar: 0g; fiber: 2g; protein: 4g; sodium: 351mg; cholesterol: 0mg

Sweet Potato Hash Browns

Skip the prepared hash browns you find in the freezer section and make them from scratch. I promise it's not that hard, and the homemade version is so much healthier and more delicious. Hash browns are a great side dish that kids love, too.

2 large sweet
potatoes, peeled

2 tablespoons olive oil

½ teaspoon sea salt

¼ teaspoon ground
black pepper

NUT-FREE
GLUTEN-FREE
DAIRY-FREE
SOY-FREE
VEGAN
KIDS LOVE IT

Active Time: 12 minutes
Total Time: 22 minutes

Yield: 4 servings
Serving size: ½ cup

1. Grate the sweet potatoes using a large cheese grater.
2. In a large skillet, heat the olive oil over medium heat. Add the sweet potatoes and cover the skillet with a lid.
3. Cook the sweet potatoes for 6 minutes. Flip them over and cook for an additional 4 minutes.
4. Turn off the heat and sprinkle with the salt and pepper. Serve hot.

Per serving: Total calories: 141; total fat: 7g; saturated fat: 1g; carbohydrates: 19g; sugar: 8g; fiber: 3g; protein: 2g; sodium: 311mg; cholesterol: 0mg

Pizza Pitas

Sometimes a snack needs to be extra-filling, and these Pizza Pitas hit the mark. I have a friend with two teenage sons who love to have these after football practice, and they're still hungry for dinner a few hours later. Although I've included this recipe in the snack section, you could always have these for dinner, especially if you're not as hungry as two teenage boys.

2 whole wheat pita breads, cut in half and split open

4 tablespoons tomato sauce

1 (5-ounce) package pepperoni slices (omit for vegetarian option)

½ cup shredded mozzarella cheese

NUT-FREE
SOY-FREE
VEGETARIAN
EXTRA QUICK
KIDS LOVE IT

Active Time: 10 minutes
Total Time: 20 minutes

Yield: 4 servings
Serving size: ½ pita

TIP: Look for whole wheat pitas in the bread section of your grocery store.

1. Preheat the oven to 350°F. Line a baking sheet with parchment paper and set aside.

2. Fill each pita half with 1 tablespoon of tomato sauce, 5 slices of pepperoni, and 2 tablespoons of cheese.

3. Lay the filled pita breads on the baking sheet. Bake for 10 minutes, or until the cheese is melted. Serve warm.

Per serving: Total calories: 305; total fat: 20g; saturated fat: 9g; carbohydrates: 19g; sugar: 2g; fiber: 3g; protein: 14g; sodium: 948mg; cholesterol:

Lemony Snap Peas

This easy vegetable dish is crisp and full of delicious lemon flavor. The peas get perfectly cooked on the stove top, and the lemon juice helps them stay nice and green. This side dish goes well with almost any main dish.

1 tablespoon olive oil

1 pound sugar snap peas

Zest and juice of 1 lemon

½ teaspoon sea salt

¼ teaspoon freshly ground black pepper

NUT-FREE
GLUTEN-FREE
DAIRY-FREE
SOY-FREE
VEGAN
EXTRA QUICK

Active Time: 10 minutes
Total Time: 13 minutes

1. In a large skillet, heat the olive oil over medium heat.

2. Add the sugar snap peas and sauté for 5 minutes, stirring occasionally. The peas will turn bright green when they are cooked through.

3. Turn off the heat and top the peas with the lemon zest and lemon juice.

4. Serve hot.

Yield: 4 servings
Serving size: One-quarter of the dish

Per serving: Total calories: 87; total fat: 4g; saturated fat: 1g; carbohydrates: 10g; sugar: 4g; fiber: 3g; protein: 3g; sodium: 304mg; cholesterol: 0mg

Cinnamon-Roasted Butternut Squash

Even though butternut squash is traditionally a fall food, I like to make this dish all year round. And, thankfully, it's usually possible to find chopped butternut squash through the year. Butternut squash has natural sugars that come out during the roasting process, making this dish taste almost as good as candy.

Nonstick cooking spray

2 pounds fresh butternut squash cubes, cut into ½-inch pieces

2 tablespoons coconut oil, warmed

1 teaspoon sea salt

½ teaspoon freshly ground black pepper

½ teaspoon ground cinnamon

NUT-FREE
GLUTEN-FREE
DAIRY-FREE
SOY-FREE
VEGAN
KIDS LOVE IT

Active Time: 10 minutes
Total Time: 30 minutes

1. Preheat the oven to 425°F. Spray a baking sheet lightly with nonstick cooking spray and set aside.

2. In a large mixing bowl, combine the butternut squash cubes, coconut oil, salt, pepper, and cinnamon, tossing to combine.

3. Pour the coated squash onto the baking sheet and bake for 20 minutes.

4. Remove the baking sheet from the oven, toss the squash, and serve it immediately.

Yield: 4 servings
Serving size: ½ cup

TIP: You can find fresh butternut squash cubes in the refrigerated section of most grocery stores. You will need to cut the cubes in half to help them cook faster.

Per serving: Total calories: 157; total fat: 7g; saturated fat: 7g; carbohydrates: 24g; sugar: 5g; fiber: 7g; protein: 2g; sodium: 10mg; cholesterol: 0mg

Paprika Pita Chips

Pita chips have gotten so popular as a tasty snack. Skip the packaged versions and make your own for a fresher taste. I like to serve these plain or with hummus on the side.

½ teaspoon smoked paprika powder

¼ teaspoon garlic powder

½ teaspoon sea salt

¼ teaspoon freshly ground black pepper

4 whole pita breads, cut into 4 wedges each

2 tablespoons olive oil, divided

NUT-FREE
DAIRY-FREE
SOY-FREE
VEGAN
KIDS LOVE IT

Active Time: 10 minutes
Total Time: 22 minutes

Yield: 4 servings
Serving size: 4 pieces

TIP: Feel free to get creative with the spices and use the ones that you like the most.

1. Preheat the oven to 400°F. Line a baking sheet with parchment paper and set aside.

2. In a small mixing bowl, combine the paprika, garlic powder, salt, and pepper.

3. Spread the pita wedges onto the baking sheet. Brush 1 tablespoon of olive oil over the top of the bread.

4. Sprinkle half of the seasoning mix over the tops of the pita wedges. Flip the wedges over and brush the other side with the remaining 1 tablespoon of olive oil and the rest of the seasoning mix.

5. Bake for 12 minutes, or until they are crisp. Let them cool for about 5 minutes, and then serve immediately.

Per serving: Total calories: 232; total fat: 9g; saturated fat: 1g; carbohydrates: 36g; sugar: 2g; fiber: 5g; protein: 6g; sodium: 631mg; cholesterol: 0mg

Garlic-Sesame Broccolini

Broccolini is a lot like broccoli, but it's longer and thinner, which makes it cook faster. I also find it to be less bitter than standard broccoli. This recipe is perfect for a quick and healthy vegetable side dish.

2 tablespoons olive oil

2 garlic cloves, minced

1 pound broccolini (about 2 bunches), cut into florets

½ teaspoon sea salt

¼ teaspoon freshly ground black pepper

1 tablespoon toasted sesame seeds

NUT-FREE
GLUTEN-FREE
DAIRY-FREE
SOY-FREE
VEGAN
EXTRA QUICK

Active Time: 10 minutes
Total Time: 14 minutes

Yield: 4 servings
Serving size: One-quarter of the dish

1. Heat the olive oil in a large skillet over medium heat. Add the garlic and broccolini, sautéing them for 6 minutes, or until the broccolini is bright green.

2. Turn off the heat and sprinkle the salt, pepper, and sesame seeds on top of the broccolini.

3. Serve hot.

Per serving: Total calories: 122; total fat: 8g; saturated fat: 1g; carbohydrates: 9g; sugar: 3g; fiber: 2g; protein: 5g; sodium: 325mg; cholesterol: 0mg

TIP: To toast the sesame seeds, heat a small non-stick skillet over low heat. Add the sesame seeds, and let them toast for about 2 minutes, being careful to not let them burn.

Cauliflower Purée

You'll never believe how much this cauliflower purée tastes like regular mashed potatoes. It's a low-carb side dish that is chock-full of fiber and nutrition. I like to serve this as an easy side dish instead of potatoes.

1 large cauliflower, cut into florets

¼ cup milk

2 tablespoons unsalted butter

½ teaspoon sea salt

¼ teaspoon freshly ground black pepper

NUT-FREE
GLUTEN-FREE
SOY-FREE
VEGETARIAN
EXTRA QUICK

Active Time: 15 minutes
Total Time: 20 minutes

Yield: 4 servings
Serving size: ⅓ cup

1. Combine the cauliflower florets and ¼ cup water in a large, microwave-safe bowl. Cover the bowl with plastic wrap and poke a few holes in the plastic.
2. Microwave for 4 minutes, or until the florets are tender.
3. Transfer the steamed cauliflower to the pitcher of a blender. Add the milk, butter, salt, and pepper. Blend for 45 seconds, or until the cauliflower is completely blended and has a creamy texture. Stop to scrape down the sides of the blender, if necessary.
4. Serve hot.

TIP: You can steam the cauliflower on the stove top instead of in the microwave, if you prefer. To do so, you'll need to steam the florets for 7 minutes over simmering water.

Per serving: Total calories: 110; total fat: 6g; saturated fat: 4g; carbohydrates: 12g; sugar: 5g; fiber: 5g; protein: 5g; sodium: 402mg; cholesterol: 16mg

Whole Wheat Parmesan Drop Biscuits

Homemade biscuits made from scratch are a healthier option than buying premade dough, because you have control over the quality of the ingredients and you can skip the preservatives. This version uses whole wheat flour for a delicious biscuit that isn't too heavy. I like to serve biscuits as a side to soups, stews, and even with salads.

Nonstick cooking spray

2 cups whole wheat flour

⅓ cup grated Parmesan cheese

4 teaspoons baking powder

½ teaspoon sea salt

4 tablespoons (½ stick) cold unsalted butter, cut into small cubes

1½ cups milk

NUT-FREE
SOY-FREE
VEGETARIAN
KIDS LOVE IT
FREEZER FRIENDLY

Active Time: 12 minutes
Total Time: 30 minutes

Yield: 12 biscuits
Serving size: 2 biscuits

TIP: Let the biscuits cool completely before storing in a zip-top bag or food container. Freeze for up to 2 months.

1. Preheat the oven to 400°F. Line a baking sheet with parchment paper and spray it lightly with nonstick cooking spray.

2. In a large mixing bowl, whisk together the flour, cheese, baking powder, and salt.

3. Add the butter, using a pastry cutter, two forks, or your fingers to cut the butter into the flour mixture. The butter should be the size of small peas.

4. Pour in the milk and stir to combine.

5. Use a large cookie scoop or ¼-cup measure to drop 12 biscuits onto the parchment paper. Bake for 14 minutes, or until the tops of the biscuits are golden brown.

6. Serve warm or at room temperature.

Per serving: Total calories: 257; total fat: 11g; saturated fat: 6g; carbohydrates: 34g; sugar: 3g; fiber: 5g; protein: 10g; sodium: 330mg; cholesterol: 29mg

Black Bean and Corn Salad

This is one of those side dishes that is perfect when you just need something quick and easy. You can serve it with baked chicken, turkey burgers, or pork chops. When I have leftovers of this dish, I like to put some sliced avocado on top and eat it for lunch the next day.

1 (15-ounce) can black beans, rinsed and drained

1 (15-ounce) can corn kernels, drained

1 cup cherry tomatoes, halved

1 red bell pepper, diced

½ red onion, diced

⅓ cup salsa

Juice of 2 limes

NUT-FREE
GLUTEN-FREE
DAIRY-FREE
SOY-FREE
VEGAN
EXTRA QUICK

Active Time: 12 minutes
Total Time: 12 minutes

1. In a medium mixing bowl, combine the black beans, corn kernels, tomatoes, bell pepper, onion, salsa, and lime juice. Stir to combine.
2. Serve at room temperature or chilled.

Yield: 4 servings
Serving size: 1 cup

Per serving: Total calories: 187; total fat: 1g; saturated fat: <1g; carbohydrates: 37g; sugar: 8g; fiber: 8g; protein: 9g; sodium: 251mg; cholesterol: 0mg

TIP: You can substitute pinto beans or red kidney beans for the black beans, if you prefer.

Ranch-Flavored Roasted Nuts

Roasted nuts are a great snack, especially when they're coated in herbs like garlic, parsley, dill, and onion. You can get creative with the types of nuts you use, but you'll need about 3 cups in total. I like the variation of textures and flavors that using cashews, almonds, and walnuts brings to this recipe.

1 cup unsalted cashews

1 cup unsalted almonds

1 cup walnuts

3 tablespoons olive oil

1 teaspoon garlic powder

1 teaspoon dried parsley flakes

1 teaspoon dried dill

1 teaspoon onion powder

1 teaspoon sea salt

GLUTEN-FREE
DAIRY-FREE
SOY-FREE
VEGAN

Active Time: 10 minutes
Total Time: 28 minutes

Yield: 9 servings
Serving size: ⅓ cup

TIP: Store any leftovers in an airtight container in the refrigerator for up to 1 month.

1. Preheat the oven to 325°F. Line a baking sheet with parchment paper and set aside.

2. In a large mixing bowl, combine the cashews, almonds, walnuts, olive oil, garlic powder, parsley, dill, onion powder, and salt. Toss to combine.

3. Pour the nuts onto the baking sheet and bake for 18 minutes, stirring the nuts every 6 minutes so they don't burn.

4. Let the nuts cool before serving.

Per serving: Total calories: 293; total fat: 27g; saturated fat: 3g; carbohydrates: 10g; sugar: 2g; fiber: 3g; protein: 8g; sodium: 262mg; cholesterol: 0mg

Balsamic Roasted Vegetables

This delicious side brings a comforting Mediterranean flair to your table and pairs well with so many main dishes. Serve it with fish, poultry, or meat to add flavor and nutrition to your protein, or toss with some tofu or tempeh for a complete, plant-based meal.

4 carrots, cut into ½-inch pieces

2 zucchini squash, cut into ½-inch slices

8 ounces button mushrooms, cut in half

1 onion, sliced

2 garlic cloves, minced

2 tablespoons olive oil

2 tablespoons balsamic vinegar

½ teaspoon sea salt

¼ teaspoon freshly ground black pepper

2 tablespoons almonds, sliced and toasted

GLUTEN-FREE
DAIRY-FREE
SOY-FREE
VEGAN

Active Time: 10 minutes
Total Time: 30 minutes

Yield: 4 servings
Serving size: ½ cup

TIP: To toast the sliced almonds, heat a small nonstick skillet over low heat. Add the almonds and let them toast for about 2 minutes, being careful to not let them burn.

1. Preheat the oven to 425°F. Line a baking sheet with parchment paper and set aside.

2. In a medium mixing bowl, combine the carrots, zucchini, mushrooms, onion, garlic, olive oil, vinegar, salt, and pepper. Toss to make sure the oil and vinegar coat all the vegetables.

3. Pour the vegetables onto the baking sheet and bake for 20 minutes, or until the vegetables have slightly browned.

4. Remove the baking sheet from the oven and sprinkle the sliced almonds on top.

5. Serve hot.

Per serving: Total calories: 147; total fat: 9g; saturated fat: 1g; carbohydrates: 16g; sugar: 7g; fiber: 4g; protein: 5g; sodium: 349mg; cholesterol: 0mg

Skillet-Baked Cornbread

I grew up eating cornbread that was made from a boxed mix. I was thrilled when I discovered this recipe for making my own homemade cornbread. It's not difficult at all to make, and the result is a wonderful, texture-rich cornbread that is perfect for serving as a satisfying side dish.

Nonstick cooking spray

1¼ cups cornmeal

1 cup buttermilk

1 cup frozen corn kernels

¾ cup whole wheat flour

2 eggs, beaten

1 tablespoon coconut sugar

1 tablespoon baking powder

1 teaspoon baking soda

1 teaspoon sea salt

NUT-FREE
GLUTEN-FREE
SOY-FREE
VEGETARIAN
KIDS LOVE IT

Active Time: 10 minutes
Total Time: 30 minutes

1. Preheat the oven to 425°F. Spray an oven-safe skillet with nonstick cooking spray and set aside.
2. In a large mixing bowl, combine the cornmeal, buttermilk, frozen corn kernels, flour, eggs, coconut sugar, baking powder, baking soda, and sea salt.
3. Bake for 20 minutes, or until the top is golden brown.
4. Let the cornbread cool for a few minutes before slicing and serving warm.

Yield: 4 servings
Serving size: One-quarter of the cornbread

TIP: You can leave out the sugar to make this recipe sugar-free.

Per serving: Total calories: 329; total fat: 5g; saturated fat: 2g; carbohydrates: 63g; sugar: 8g; fiber: 7g; protein: 13g; sodium: 1,1015mg; cholesterol: 96mg

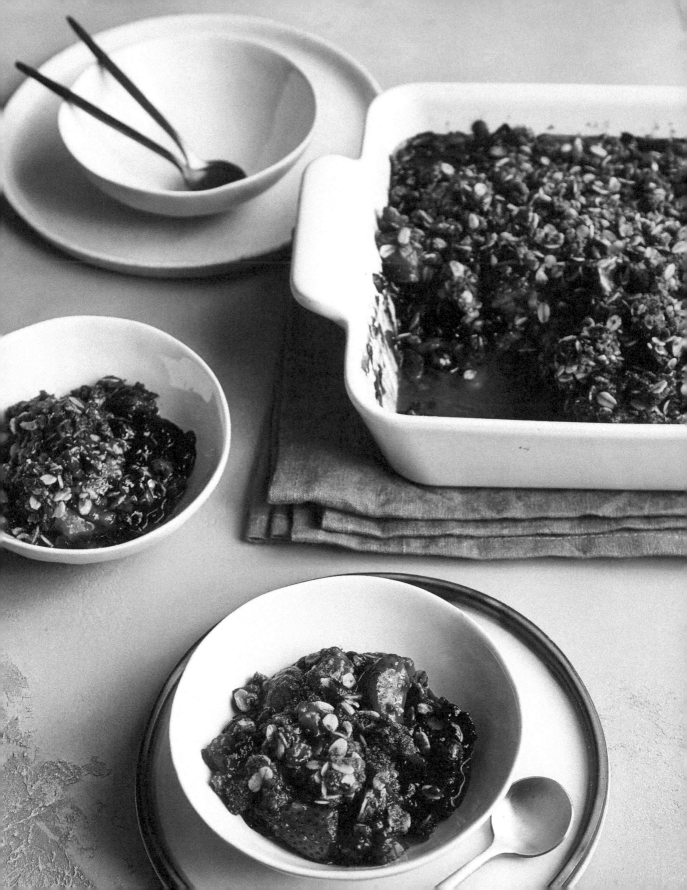

Desserts

Healthy Berry Cobbler with Oat Topping

No-Bake Sunflower Butter Balls

These Sunflower Butter Balls are a great snack or dessert. Sometimes I even have them after a workout for a quick-and-easy way to refuel. Sunflower butter tastes a lot like peanut butter and is a great nut-free option.

1½ cup rolled oats (for gluten-free option, use gluten-free oats)

½ cup sunflower seed butter, at room temperature

¼ cup maple syrup

NUT-FREE
GLUTEN-FREE
DAIRY-FREE
SOY-FREE
VEGAN
EXTRA QUICK
KIDS LOVE IT
FREEZER FRIENDLY

Active Time: 10 minutes
Total Time: 20 minutes

Yield: 2 dozen balls
Serving size: 2 balls

1. Put the oats in the pitcher of your food processor or blender. Process or blend on high for 30 seconds, or until blended into flour.

2. Add the sunflower seed butter and maple syrup and process or blend for an additional 45 seconds, or until the mixture comes together.

3. Pour the mixture into a medium mixing bowl and use your hands to form 24 balls, using about 1 tablespoon of dough per ball.

4. Store the balls in a glass bowl with a lid for up to 1 week in the refrigerator. Serve them cold.

TIPS: Look for sunflower seed butter without any added sugar.

Store any leftovers in a zip-top bag in the freezer for up to 2 months. Defrost the balls in the fridge before serving.

Per serving (2 balls): Total calories: 121; total fat: 6g; saturated fat: 1g; carbohydrates: 14g; sugar: 5g; fiber: 2g; protein: 4g; sodium: 41mg; cholesterol: 0mg

Peanut Butter Blossoms

These flourless peanut butter cookies with a melty chocolate center are absolutely delicious. They're both grain-free and gluten-free, with the rich flavor of peanut butter. I like to serve these during the holidays because everyone seems to love them so much.

1 cup natural peanut butter, at room temperature

1 cup coconut sugar

1 egg, beaten

1 teaspoon vanilla extract

24 chocolate chunks or chocolate drops (for dairy-free option, use vegan chocolate chunks)

GLUTEN-FREE
DAIRY-FREE
SOY-FREE
VEGETARIAN
KIDS LOVE IT

Active Time: 10 minutes
Total Time: 25 minutes

Yield: 2 dozen cookies
Serving size: 2 cookies

TIPS: Look for vegan chocolate chunks in the baking section of your grocery store.

Look for peanut butter brands that have no added sugar or oil to make this an extra-healthy treat.

1. Preheat the oven to 350°F. Line a baking sheet with parchment paper and set aside.

2. In a medium bowl, combine the peanut butter, sugar, egg, and vanilla. Stir to combine.

3. Use your hands to form 24 balls from the dough, using about 1 tablespoon of dough per ball.

4. Lay the balls on the baking sheet about 1 inch apart.

5. Bake the cookies for 10 minutes. Remove the baking sheet from the oven and immediately press a chocolate chunk or chocolate drop into the center of each cookie.

6. Let the cookies cool for 5 minutes before serving.

Per serving (2 cookies): Total calories: 238; total fat: 14g; saturated fat: 4g; carbohydrates: 26g; sugar: 23g; fiber: 2g; protein: 7g; sodium: 113mg; cholesterol: 18mg

Edible Chocolate Chip Cookie Dough

You know how you're not supposed to eat raw cookie dough, but you always want to? Now you can, with this egg-free version made from almond flour. You can get creative and add in sprinkles or white chocolate chips.

1½ cups almond flour

¼ cup maple syrup

2 tablespoons coconut oil, melted

1 tablespoon vanilla extract

¼ teaspoon sea salt

⅓ cup dairy-free chocolate chips

GLUTEN-FREE
DAIRY-FREE
SOY-FREE
VEGAN
EXTRA QUICK
KIDS LOVE IT

Active Time: 10 minutes
Total Time: 10 minutes

1. In a medium mixing bowl, combine the almond flour, maple syrup, coconut oil, vanilla, and sea salt. Stir to combine well.

2. Add the chocolate chips and stir the mixture once more.

3. Serve at room temperature or chilled.

Per serving: Total calories: 459; total fat: 34g; saturated fat: 12g; carbohydrates: 34g; sugar: 22g; fiber: 6g; protein: 10g; sodium: 147mg; cholesterol: 0mg

Yield: 4 servings
Serving size: ⅓ cup

TIPS: You can find dairy-free chocolate chips in the baking aisle of most grocery stores for a vegan take on this treat.

Store any leftovers in an airtight container in the refrigerator for up to a week.

Raspberry Chocolate Chia Pudding

Chia seeds are a magical ingredient that soaks up whatever liquid you mix them with. They're also a nutritional powerhouse, containing fiber, protein, and important vitamins and minerals. Chia seeds are the base of this easy pudding recipe, which doubles as a healthy dessert and tasty snack.

1¼ cups unsweetened plain almond milk

¼ cup maple syrup

6 tablespoons chia seeds

2 tablespoons cocoa powder

1 teaspoon vanilla extract

½ cup frozen raspberries

GLUTEN-FREE
DAIRY-FREE
SOY-FREE
VEGAN

Active Time: 10 minutes
Total Time: 25 minutes

Yield: **2 servings**
Serving size: ½ cup

1. Combine the almond milk, maple syrup, chia seeds, cocoa powder, vanilla, and frozen raspberries in the pitcher of a blender. Blend on high for 45 seconds until the ingredients are well combined.

2. Pour the mixture into two glasses and put them in the refrigerator for 15 minutes to set.

3. Serve this cold or at room temperature.

TIP: Use whatever frozen berry you like the most in this recipe, including strawberries or blueberries.

Per serving: Total calories: 344; total fat: 12g; saturated fat: 0g; carbohydrates: 50g; sugar: 26g; fiber: 19g; protein: 11g; sodium: 131mg; cholesterol: 0mg

Pineapple Coconut Fruit Salad

This easy dessert has the flavor of a piña colada because of the pineapple and coconut. While I am usually partial to chocolate desserts, I love to make this fruit salad to take to parties or potlucks. With no added sugars, this is a great dessert to enjoy when you're trying to eat healthier.

1 (20-ounce) can pineapple chunks, with the juice

1 banana, sliced

1 pint strawberries, hulled and halved

1 cup blueberries

1 cup green grapes, halved

¼ cup shredded, unsweetened dried coconut

Juice of 2 limes

NUT-FREE
GLUTEN-FREE
DAIRY-FREE
SOY-FREE
VEGAN
EXTRA QUICK
KIDS LOVE IT

Active Time: 12 minutes
Total Time: 12 minutes

1. In a medium mixing bowl, combine the pineapple, banana, strawberries, blueberries, grapes, coconut, and lime juice and stir.

2. Serve chilled or at room temperature.

Per serving: Total calories: 87; total fat: 2g; saturated fat: 1g; carbohydrates: 18g; sugar: 14g; fiber: 2g; protein: 1g; sodium: 3mg; cholesterol: 0mg

Yield: 10 servings
Serving size: ½ cup

TIP: You can use whatever combination of fresh fruits you like, but you will need a total of about 5 cups. Store any leftovers in the refrigerator for up to 4 days.

Single-Serving Chocolate Mug Cake

This recipe is perfect for those days when you don't want to bake a whole cake, but you're craving a single-serving chocolate treat. This recipe is grain-free, gluten-free, and dairy-free, but it amazingly has the consistency of real cake.

¼ cup almond flour

2 tablespoons cocoa powder

2 tablespoons maple syrup

1 teaspoon coconut oil

1 teaspoon vanilla extract

1 egg, beaten

1 tablespoon dairy-free chocolate chips

GLUTEN-FREE
DAIRY-FREE
SOY-FREE
VEGETARIAN
EXTRA QUICK

Active Time: 5 minutes
Total Time: 10 minutes

Yield: 1 serving
Serving size: 1 mug

TIP: Use a 10- or 12-ounce mug for this recipe.

1. In a medium, microwave-safe bowl, combine the almond flour, cocoa powder, maple syrup, coconut oil, vanilla, and the egg. Whisk the ingredients together until the mixture is smooth and pour into a coffee mug.

2. Microwave for 2 minutes, or until the cake has risen.

3. Remove the mug from the microwave. Sprinkle the chocolate chips on top so they can start to melt. Let the cake cool for 3 minutes before serving it warm.

Per serving: Total calories: 491; total fat: 29g; saturated fat: 9g; carbohydrates: 49g; sugar: 34g; fiber: 5g; protein: 15g; sodium: 85mg; cholesterol: 191mg

Grain-Free Chocolate Chip Cookies

These chocolate chip cookies are made grain-free and gluten-free using almond flour instead of wheat flour. The texture of the cookies is slightly crisper than regular cookies, and the crispy texture makes them a light treat perfect for dunking. I like to freeze half of the batch for a later date, and to keep me from eating them all in one sitting.

2 cups almond flour

¼ cup coconut sugar

½ teaspoon baking soda

¼ teaspoon sea salt

½ cup coconut oil, warmed

1 egg, beaten

1 tablespoon vanilla extract

1 cup dairy-free chocolate chips

GLUTEN-FREE
DAIRY-FREE
SOY-FREE
VEGAN
KIDS LOVE IT
FREEZER FRIENDLY

Active Time: 10 minutes
Total Time: 30 minutes

Yield: **2 dozen cookies**
Serving size: **2 cookies**

TIP: To freeze any leftovers, let the cookies cool completely. Put them in a zip-top bag and freeze them for up to 2 months.

1. Preheat the oven to 350°F. Line a baking sheet with parchment paper and set aside.

2. In a large mixing bowl, combine the almond flour, sugar, baking soda, and sea salt. Stir to combine.

3. Add the coconut oil, egg, and vanilla and stir to combine.

4. Stir in the chocolate chips.

5. Use your hands to form 24 tablespoon-size balls and lay them on the cookie sheet. Bake them for 12 minutes, or until the cookies have turned golden brown.

6. Remove the baking sheet from the oven and let the cookies cool for about 5 minutes before serving.

Per serving (2 cookies): Total calories: 300; total fat: 25g; saturated fat: 12g; carbohydrates: 20g; sugar: 15g; fiber: 2g; protein: 6g; sodium: 120mg; cholesterol: 22mg

Chocolate No-Bake Cookies

I remember making a version of these no-bake cookies with my mom as a kid in the Midwest during the summer. It was just too hot to turn on the oven, so these were a great alternative. This recipe is vegan and gluten-free, with lots of chewy texture.

1 banana, mashed

¼ cup coconut oil, melted

½ cup almond butter, at room temperature

3 cups rolled oats (for gluten-free option, use gluten-free oats)

⅓ cup coconut sugar

¼ cup cocoa powder

¼ cup unsweetened plain almond milk

½ teaspoon vanilla extract

¼ teaspoon sea salt

GLUTEN-FREE
DAIRY-FREE
SOY-FREE
VEGAN
KIDS LOVE IT
FREEZER FRIENDLY

Active Time: 10 minutes
Total Time: 25 minutes

Yield: **2 dozen cookies**
Serving size: **2 cookies**

TIP: Store the cookies in the refrigerator for up to 1 week. Alternately, put the cookies in a zip-top bag and store them in the freezer for up to 2 months. Let the cookies defrost in the refrigerator for a few hours before consuming.

1. Line a baking sheet with parchment paper and set it aside.
2. In a large mixing bowl, combine the banana, coconut oil, and almond butter. Stir to combine.
3. Add the oats, coconut sugar, cocoa powder, almond milk, vanilla, and salt and stir to combine.
4. Use a tablespoon to form 24 cookies from the dough, laying each one on the parchment paper about 1 inch apart. Put the baking sheet in the refrigerator for 15 minutes so the cookies can firm up before eating.

Per serving (2 cookies): Total calories: 212; total fat: 12g; saturated fat: 5g; carbohydrates: 24g; sugar: 8g; fiber: 4g; protein: 5g; sodium: 54mg; cholesterol: 0mg

Ginger Molasses Cookies

This holiday cookie favorite is made with whole wheat flour, which adds fiber and nutrition. The molasses and ginger are the keys to making this cookie taste like gingerbread. You're going to want to make these throughout the whole year and not just at the holidays.

4 tablespoons (½ stick) unsalted butter, at room temperature

¾ cup coconut sugar, divided

¼ cup blackstrap molasses

1 egg, beaten

1¾ cups whole wheat flour

2 teaspoons baking soda

2 teaspoons ground ginger

1 teaspoon ground cinnamon

¼ teaspoon sea salt

NUT-FREE
SOY-FREE
VEGETARIAN
KIDS LOVE IT
FREEZER FRIENDLY

Active Time: 15 minutes
Total Time: 25 minutes

Yield: 2 dozen cookies
Serving size: 2 cookies

TIP: To freeze any leftovers, let the cookies cool completely. Put them in a zip-top bag and freeze them up to 2 months.

1. Preheat the oven to 350°F. Line a baking sheet with parchment paper and set aside.

2. In a large mixing bowl, combine the butter, ½ cup of coconut sugar, the molasses, and egg. Stir to combine.

3. Add the flour, baking soda, ground ginger, cinnamon, and salt to the mixing bowl. Stir to combine.

4. Use your hands to form the dough into 24 balls, using about 1 tablespoon of dough per ball.

5. Put the remaining ¼ cup of sugar on a small plate. Roll each dough ball over the sugar and then lay the balls onto the baking sheet. Use the palm of your hand to press the balls into a cookie shape.

6. Bake them for 10 minutes. Let the cookies cool slightly before serving.

Per serving (2 cookies): Total calories: 162; total fat: 5g; saturated fat: 3g; carbohydrates: 29g; sugar: 12g; fiber: 2g; protein: 3g; sodium: 295mg; cholesterol: 26mg

Peanut Butter and Banana Oat Bars

These bars are sweet enough to have for dessert, but they also make an excellent snack. The ripe bananas add most of the natural sweetness, with the maple syrup and chocolate chips adding just a bit more. This healthy dessert is a winner with both kids and grown-ups.

Nonstick cooking spray

2 bananas

1 cup rolled oats (for gluten-free option, use gluten-free oats)

½ cup natural peanut butter, at room temperature

1 egg, beaten

2 tablespoons maple syrup

1 teaspoon vanilla extract

½ teaspoon baking soda

½ teaspoon ground cinnamon

¼ cup dairy-free chocolate chips

GLUTEN-FREE
DAIRY-FREE
SOY-FREE
VEGETARIAN
KIDS LOVE IT
FREEZER FRIENDLY

Active Time: 10 minutes

Total Time: 30 minutes

Yield: 2 dozen cookies
Serving size: 2 cookies

TIP: Look for peanut butter brands that have no added sugars or oils.

1. Preheat the oven to 375°F. Spray an 8-by-8-inch square baking dish with nonstick cooking spray and set aside.

2. Put the bananas in a medium mixing bowl. Use a fork to mash them well.

3. Add the oats, peanut butter, egg, maple syrup, vanilla, baking soda, and cinnamon. Stir to combine.

4. Pour the mixture into the baking dish and use your hands or a spatula to press the mixture evenly into the pan.

5. Top the mixture with the chocolate chips. Bake for 20 minutes, or until the top of the mixture has turned a golden brown. Let the bars cool slightly before slicing and serving.

Per serving (2 cookies): Total calories: 145; total fat: 8g; saturated fat: 2g; carbohydrates: 17g; sugar: 8g; fiber: 2g; protein: 5g; sodium: 66mg; cholesterol: 17mg

Pumpkin-Oatmeal Chocolate Chip Cookies

Nobody will ever believe that these cookies have vegetables in them. The canned pumpkin helps displace some of the oil, while adding nutrition and fiber. Don't worry, these healthy cookies are still absolutely delicious.

1 cup whole wheat flour

1 cup coconut sugar

¾ cup rolled oats

⅓ cup dairy-free chocolate chips

1 teaspoon ground cinnamon

½ teaspoon baking soda

¼ teaspoon sea salt

¾ cup canned pumpkin

¼ cup coconut oil, melted

1 egg, beaten

1 teaspoon vanilla extract

NUT-FREE
DAIRY-FREE
SOY-FREE
VEGETARIAN
KIDS LOVE IT
FREEZER FRIENDLY

Active Time: 10 minutes
Total Time: 30 minutes

Yield: 2 dozen cookies
Serving size: 2 cookies

TIPS: Use canned pumpkin with no other ingredients other than pumpkin. (Do not use canned pumpkin pie mix, which is a different product.)

To freeze any leftovers, let the cookies cool completely. Put them to a zip-top bag and freeze them for up to 2 months.

1. Preheat the oven to 350°F. Line a baking sheet with parchment paper and set aside.

2. In a large mixing bowl, combine the flour, sugar, oats, chocolate chips, cinnamon, baking soda, and salt. Stir to combine.

3. In a medium mixing bowl, combine the canned pumpkin, coconut oil, egg, and vanilla.

4. Pour the wet ingredients into the dry ingredients and stir to combine.

5. Drop a rounded tablespoon of the batter onto the parchment paper, leaving about 1 inch of space between each cookie.

6. Bake for 15 minutes, or until the cookies have turned golden brown. Let cool for a few minutes before serving.

Per serving (2 cookies): Total calories: 193; total fat: 7g; saturated fat: 5g; carbohydrates: 32g; sugar: 20g; fiber: 2g; protein: 3g; sodium: 112mg; cholesterol: 18mg

Healthy Berry Cobbler with Oat Topping

This berry dessert recipe is a favorite of mine at any time of year, but especially in the spring and summer, when fresh berries are available. The crumble is full of texture, almost like an oatmeal cookie. Plus, berries are a great source of antioxidants and fiber, making this a nutritious delight.

Nonstick cooking spray

¾ cup whole wheat flour

¾ cup quick-cook oats

¾ cup coconut sugar

½ teaspoon cinnamon

¼ teaspoon sea salt

6 tablespoons cold unsalted butter, cubed

1 pound strawberries, hulled and halved

1 cup blueberries

Juice of 1 lemon

3 tablespoons cornstarch

NUT-FREE
SOY-FREE
VEGETARIAN

Active Time: 10 minutes
Total Time: 30 minutes

Yield: 8 servings
Serving size: ⅓ cup

TIP: You can use frozen berries for this recipe, but you will need to defrost them in the refrigerator overnight or in the microwave before baking. There is no need to drain the juice.

1. Preheat the oven to 375°F. Spray an 8-by-8-inch square baking dish with nonstick cooking spray and set aside.

2. In a medium mixing bowl, combine the flour, oats, sugar, cinnamon, and salt. Stir to combine.

3. Add the butter, using a pastry cutter, two forks, or your fingers to cut the butter into the flour mixture. The butter should be the size of small peas.

4. In a separate, medium mixing bowl, combine the strawberries, blueberries, lemon juice, and corn-starch. Toss to combine.

5. Pour the berry mixture into the bottom of the baking dish and use a spatula to spread it into a flat layer.

6. Pour the flour-and-oat mixture over the berries, and use your spatula to spread it evenly across the top.

7. Bake for 20 minutes. Serve warm.

Per serving: Total calories: 251; total fat: 10g; saturated fat: 6g; carbohydrates: 41g; sugar: 23g; fiber: 4g; protein: 3g; sodium: 136mg; cholesterol: 23mg

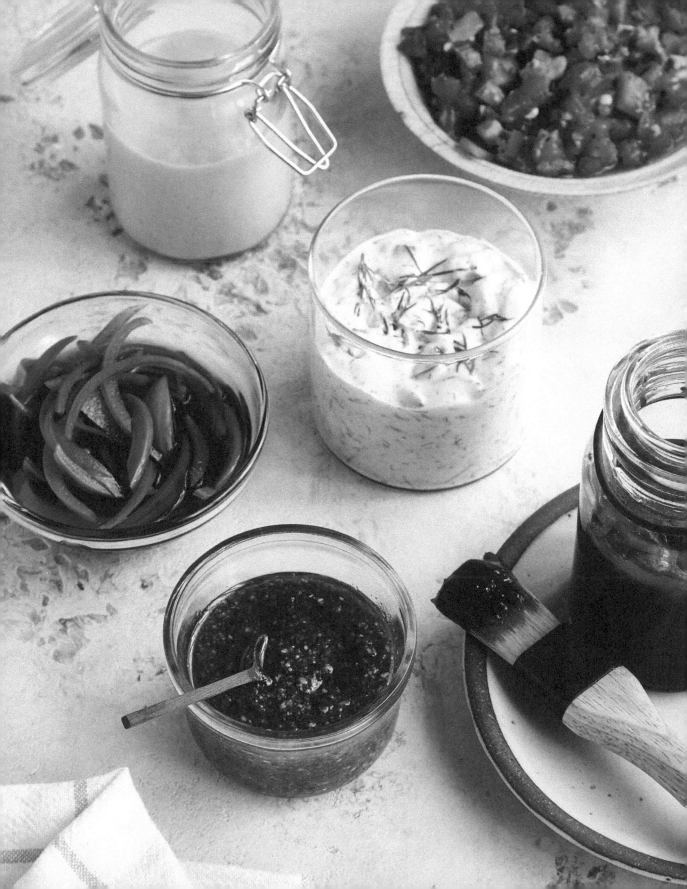

CHAPTER TEN

Basics & Extras

Baked Potatoes

It can take more than an hour to make baked potatoes in the oven. This recipe uses both the microwave and the oven to speed up the process. I like to serve baked potatoes as a hearty side dish to go with my Chipotle-Baked Salmon (page 62) or Panfried Honey Mustard Pork Chops (page 99).

---

4 small russet potatoes

1. Preheat the oven to 425°F.

2. Scrub the potatoes and pat them dry. Prick each potato with a fork several times all around.

3. Put the potatoes on a microwave-safe plate and microwave on high for 6 minutes.

4. Remove the plate from the microwave carefully so as not to burn yourself, and transfer the potatoes to a baking dish.

5. Bake the potatoes for 20 minutes. Cut them open and let them cool for a few minutes before serving.

Per serving: Total calories: 110; total fat: 0g; saturated fat: 0g; carbohydrates: 26g; sugar: 1g; fiber: 2g; protein: 3g; sodium: 0mg; cholesterol: 0mg

NUT-FREE
GLUTEN-FREE
DAIRY-FREE
SOY-FREE
VEGAN

Active Time: 10 minutes
Total Time: 30 minutes

Yield: **4 servings**
Serving size: **1 potato**

Cooked Brown Lentils

I like to make a batch of cooked brown lentils to have on hand when planning meals for the week. You can always throw them on top of a salad or into soup to add great plant-based protein and texture. Cooked lentils can even be their own meal by serving them with a vinaigrette and sliced avocado on top.

---

1 cup brown lentils
1 bay leaf

3 cups filtered water

NUT-FREE
GLUTEN-FREE
DAIRY-FREE
SOY-FREE
VEGAN

Active Time: 10 minutes
Total Time: 28 minutes

Yield: 2½ cups
Serving size: ½ cup

TIP: Cooked lentils can be stored in an airtight container in the refrigerator for up to 1 week or in the freezer for up to 2 months.

1. Put the lentils in a colander and pick through them to remove any debris.
2. Rinse them well and put them in a medium saucepan, along with the bay leaf.
3. Add the water and bring the mixture to a boil. Turn the heat to low, cover the pan, and let them simmer for 18 minutes. The lentils should absorb most of the water and should be fairly soft when they are fully cooked, but will still retain their shape.
4. Turn off the heat, and remove and discard the bay leaf.
5. Serve immediately or store to serve later.

Per serving: Total calories: 120; total fat: 1g; saturated fat: 0g; carbohydrates: 20g; sugar: 2g; fiber: 10g; protein: 10g; sodium: 4mg; cholesterol: 0mg

Easiest Homemade Guacamole

Skip the packaged guacamole and make it at home. It's one of the easiest side dishes you can make, and it goes with almost everything. I like to serve it with any of my Mexican-inspired dishes, such as my Loaded Chicken and Black Bean Nachos (page 90) or my Taco Salad Beef Skillet (page 107). Or, if I'm really short on time, I'll just combine some shredded lettuce and cooked chicken cubes in a bowl with a dollop of this guacamole on top and call it a meal.

3 avocados, halved and pitted

2 tablespoons chopped fresh cilantro

1 garlic clove, minced

Juice of 2 limes

½ teaspoon sea salt

¼ teaspoon freshly ground black pepper

NUT-FREE
GLUTEN-FREE
DAIRY-FREE
SOY-FREE
VEGAN
EXTRA QUICK

Active Time: 10 minutes
Total Time: 10 minutes

Yield: 6 servings
Serving size: ¼ cup

1. Use a spoon to scoop out the flesh from the avocados into a small mixing bowl.

2. Add the cilantro, garlic, lime juice, salt, and pepper. Stir to combine.

3. Serve chilled or at room temperature.

Per serving: Total calories: 149; total fat: 13g; saturated fat: 2g; carbohydrates: 8g; sugar: 1g; fiber: 6g; protein: 2g; sodium: 201mg; cholesterol: 0mg

TIP: If you don't like the flavor of cilantro, you can just leave it out or use fresh, chopped flat-leaf parsley instead.

Pico de Gallo

Fresh pico de gallo is so easy to make and adds authentic flavor to any Mexican-inspired dish. The combination of flavors is also perfect for adding freshness and a spicy kick. I like to serve it with my Vegan Tempeh Tacos (page 53), Easy Fish Tacos (page 74), and Loaded Chicken and Black Bean Nachos (page 90).

4 large tomatoes, diced

1 jalapeño pepper, seeded and finely diced

½ onion, diced

½ cup chopped fresh cilantro

Juice of 2 limes

½ teaspoon sea salt

NUT-FREE
GLUTEN-FREE
DAIRY-FREE
SOY-FREE
VEGAN
EXTRA QUICK

Active Time: 10 minutes
Total Time: 10 minutes

1. Combine the tomatoes, jalapeño, onion, cilantro, lime juice, and salt in a medium mixing bowl. Stir to combine.

2. Serve at room temperature or chilled.

Per serving: Total calories: 35; total fat: <1g; saturated fat: <1g; carbohydrates: 7g; sugar: 4g; fiber: 2g; protein: 1g; sodium: 206mg; cholesterol: 0mg

Yield: 6 servings
Serving size: ¼ cup

TIP: Leave out the jalapeño pepper if you don't like spicy foods. Store any leftovers in an airtight container in the refrigerator for up to 4 days.

Tzatziki Yogurt Sauce

This creamy Mediterranean condiment is one of my favorite toppings for baked fish, chicken, and even salads. Because of its cooling properties, it's also great to serve with spicy foods, such as my Mediterranean Beef Bowl (page 108). Even kids like this flavorful sauce.

1½ cups Greek yogurt

1 cucumber, grated

Juice of 1 lemon

1 teaspoon dried dill

½ teaspoon sea salt

¼ teaspoon freshly ground black pepper

¼ teaspoon garlic powder

NUT-FREE
GLUTEN-FREE
SOY-FREE
VEGETARIAN
EXTRA QUICK
KIDS LOVE IT

Active Time: 12 minutes
Total Time: 12 minutes

---

1. In a medium mixing bowl, combine the yogurt, cucumber, lemon juice, dill, salt, pepper, and garlic powder. Stir to combine.

2. Serve chilled or at room temperature.

Yield: 8 servings
Serving size: ½ cup

Per serving: Total calories: 48; total fat: 3g; saturated fat: 2g; carbohydrates: 5g; sugar: 4g; fiber: <1g; protein: 2g; sodium: 175mg; cholesterol: 9mg

Blender Pesto

Homemade pesto is one of my favorite things to make in spring and summer, when fresh basil is abundant. You just can't beat the flavor and freshness of this homemade version. I like to serve it with baked chicken or fish, including my Pesto-Baked Salmon and Vegetables (page 70).

2 cups fresh basil, tightly packed

½ cup olive oil

Juice of 1 lemon

1 garlic clove, minced

¼ cup pine nuts

¼ cup grated Parmesan cheese (omit for vegan option)

¼ teaspoon sea salt

GLUTEN-FREE
SOY-FREE
VEGAN

Active Time: 10 minutes
Total Time: 30 minutes

1. In the pitcher of a blender, combine the basil, olive oil, lemon juice, garlic, pine nuts, cheese, and salt. Blend on for about 45 seconds, or until it is well combined.

2. Serve chilled or at room temperature.

Yield: 4 servings
Serving size: 2 tablespoons

TIP: If you don't have enough basil for 2 cups, you can mix in baby spinach.

Per serving: Total calories: 334; total fat: 35g; saturated fat: 5g; carbohydrates: 4g; sugar: 1g; fiber: 1g; protein: 4g; sodium: 263mg; cholesterol: 5mg

Quick Vegetable Broth

I usually buy boxed vegetable broth to keep in my pantry, but making a homemade veggie broth is easier than you might think. It's a great way to save money and use up any of your leftover vegetable scraps, such as the ends of carrots or celery sticks. If you have extra time, you can let the broth simmer for up to 2 hours. Otherwise, just 20 minutes will be enough time for a rich flavor to develop.

4 medium carrots, peeled and chopped into 1-inch chunks

4 celery stalks, chopped

1 onion, chopped

4 garlic cloves, chopped

1 bay leaf

1 sprig fresh thyme, rosemary, or oregano

NUT-FREE
GLUTEN-FREE
DAIRY-FREE
SOY-FREE
VEGAN

Active Time: 10 minutes
Total Time: 30 minutes

Yield: 8 cups
Serving size: 2 cups

1. In a large pot, combine 8 cups of water with the carrots, celery, onion, garlic, and herbs. Bring to a boil.

2. Turn the heat to low, cover the pot, and let simmer for 20 minutes.

3. Strain the broth into a large bowl, discarding the cooked vegetables. Use the broth immediately or let cool before dividing up and storing in the refrigerator or freezer.

TIP: You can keep the broth in the refrigerator for up to 1 week. Freeze any leftovers in airtight containers for up to 2 months. Defrost in the refrigerator before using.

Per serving: Total calories: 17; total fat: <1g; saturated fat: <1g; carbohydrates: 4g; sugar: 0g; fiber: 1g; protein: 1g; sodium: 17mg; cholesterol: 0mg

Herbed Cubed Chicken

Having cooked chicken on hand is a great way to meal prep for the week. This chicken recipe is super versatile and can be used in a variety of dishes, including Curry Chicken Salad (page 30) and Waldorf Chicken Salad with Chopped Apples, Grapes, and Walnuts (page 31). Or, you can just toss the cooked chicken on top of cooked rice, pasta, or vegetables, and serve it with a splash of balsamic vinegar for a super-easy meal.

¼ cup olive oil

1 pound boneless, skinless chicken breasts, cut into 1-inch cubes

1 garlic clove, minced

½ teaspoon dried oregano

½ teaspoon dried thyme

½ teaspoon sea salt

¼ teaspoon freshly ground black pepper

NUT-FREE
GLUTEN-FREE
DAIRY-FREE
SOY-FREE

Active Time: 10 minutes
Total Time: 30 minutes

1. In a large nonstick skillet, heat the oil over medium heat. Add the chicken and stir to coat with the oil.

2. Add the garlic, oregano, thyme, salt, and pepper and stir again to combine.

3. Cover the skillet with a lid and let the chicken cook for 8 minutes, or until the center is no longer pink, stirring occasionally to keep it from burning.

4. Serve immediately or store for later use.

Per serving: Total calories: 232; total fat: 16g; saturated fat: 2g; carbohydrates: 1g; sugar: 0g; fiber: <1g; protein: 23g; sodium: 471mg; cholesterol: 65mg

Yield: 4 servings
Serving size: ½ cup

TIP: To save the leftovers to use later, transfer the chicken to an airtight container and store in the refrigerator for up to 4 days. You can eat this dish chilled or reheated on the stove top or in the microwave.

Honey Mustard Dressing

Honey mustard dressing was my favorite growing up, and I still love its sweet-and-sour flavor profile. This dressing is a great way to introduce kids to salads. You can even use this dressing as a dip for carrot or celery sticks to get them to eat more fresh vegetables.

½ cup Greek yogurt

¼ cup olive oil

¼ cup Dijon mustard

⅓ cup honey

1 tablespoon apple cider vinegar

Juice of 1 lemon

¼ teaspoon sea salt

¼ teaspoon freshly ground black pepper

NUT-FREE
GLUTEN-FREE
SOY-FREE
VEGETARIAN
EXTRA QUICK
KIDS LOVE IT

Active Time: 10 minutes
Total Time: 10 minutes

Yield: 8 servings
Serving size: 3 tablespoons

1. In a medium mixing bowl, whisk together the yogurt, olive oil, mustard, honey, vinegar, lemon juice, salt, and pepper in a medium mixing bowl.

2. Store the dressing in the refrigerator in an airtight container for up to 1 week.

Per serving: Total calories: 125; total fat: 8g; saturated fat: 2g; carbohydrates: 13g; sugar: 13g; fiber: <1g; protein: 1g; sodium: 263mg; cholesterol: 3mg

Quick-Pickled Onions

Tart pickled onions are a great side dish or condiment to serve with main dish recipes. The onions kick up the flavor up a notch and have a nice, crunchy texture. I like to serve them with my Beef Burgers with Portobello Buns (page 101), Barbecue Meatloaf Muffins (page 102), and any other dish that can stand up to the tart flavor.

1 onion, thinly sliced

½ cup white wine vinegar

½ cup apple cider vinegar

2 tablespoons sugar

1½ teaspoons sea salt

1 teaspoon dried oregano

1 bay leaf

NUT-FREE
GLUTEN-FREE
DAIRY-FREE
SOY-FREE
VEGAN

Active Time: 10 minutes
Total Time: 30 minutes

Yield: 4 servings
Serving size: 2 tablespoons

TIP: You can store these quick-pickled onions in an airtight container in the refrigerator for up to 1 week.

1. Put the onions in the bottom of a heat-safe, quart-size jar or vessel with a lid.

2. In a medium saucepan over high heat, combine ½ cup water with the vinegars, sugar, salt, oregano, and bay leaf. Bring to a boil, then turn the heat to low and simmer for 3 minutes, stirring occasionally. Turn off heat, and allow the mixture to cool briefly to avoid breaking the jar.

3. Pour the mixture carefully over the onions in the jar.

4. Let the jar sit on the countertop to cool for at least 15 minutes.

5. Use a fork to pull out the onions from the liquid in the jar to serve.

Per serving: Total calories: 42; total fat: <1g; saturated fat: 0g; carbohydrates: 9g; sugar: 8g; fiber: 1g; protein: <1g; sodium: 873mg; cholesterol: 0mg

Easy Homemade Barbecue Sauce

Most barbecue sauces are made with refined sugars, but this recipe uses dates instead. Dates are a whole food full of fiber and minerals and are the perfect addition to this homemade sauce. I like to make a batch and use it on my Barbecue Meatloaf Muffins (page 102) and as a condiment to baked chicken or steak.

1 cup balsamic vinegar

1 (6-ounce) can tomato paste

6 Medjool dates, pitted

2 tablespoons Dijon mustard

2 tablespoons reduced-sodium tamari

½ teaspoon garlic powder

½ teaspoon sea salt

¼ teaspoon freshly ground black pepper

NUT-FREE
GLUTEN-FREE
DAIRY-FREE
VEGAN

Active Time: 10 minutes
Total Time: 30 minutes

1. In a medium saucepan, combine ½ cup water with the vinegar, tomato paste, dates, mustard, tamari, garlic powder, salt, and pepper. Bring it to a simmer over medium heat and cook for 3 minutes.

2. Turn off the heat and transfer the mixture to the pitcher of a blender. Carefully blend the mixture on high for 30 seconds, or until the dates have incorporated into the sauce.

3. Pour the mixture into a jar. Use immediately or store in the refrigerator for up to 1 week.

Yield: 4 servings
Serving size: 2 tablespoons

TIP: Be extra careful when blending hot liquids. I always like to put a dish towel over the top of the lid in case any of the liquid escapes during blending.

Per serving: Total calories: 183; total fat: <1g; saturated fat: 0g; carbohydrates: 44g; sugar: 29g; fiber: 4g; protein: 4g; sodium: 1,177mg; cholesterol: 0mg

Golden Rice Pilaf

This is one of my favorite side dishes because it goes with almost everything. Turmeric provides a natural yellow food coloring, and the addition of raisins and almonds gives this rice dish so much great texture. Kids love it because of its slightly sweet flavor.

1 tablespoon olive oil

1 shallot, diced

1 garlic clove, minced

1 cup white long-grain rice, rinsed

2 cups reduced-sodium vegetable broth

1 teaspoon ground turmeric

¼ cup sliced almonds

¼ cup raisins

1 tablespoon unsweetened shredded coconut

Juice of 1 lemon

½ teaspoon sea salt

¼ teaspoon freshly ground black pepper

GLUTEN-FREE
DAIRY-FREE
SOY-FREE
VEGAN
KIDS LOVE IT

Active Time: 10 minutes
Total Time: 28 minutes

Yield: 4 servings
Serving size: 1 cup

1. In a large saucepan, heat the oil over medium heat. Add the shallot and garlic and sauté for 3 minutes. Stir occasionally to keep them from burning.

2. Add the rice, broth, and turmeric and turn the heat to high. Bring to a boil, then turn the heat to low, cover, and let simmer for 18 minutes, until the rice has absorbed most of the liquid.

3. Stir in the almonds, raisins, coconut, lemon juice, salt, and pepper. Serve hot.

Per serving: Total calories: 286; total fat: 8g; saturated fat: 2g; carbohydrates: 50g; sugar: 8g; fiber: 3g; protein: 5g; sodium: 365mg; cholesterol: 0mg

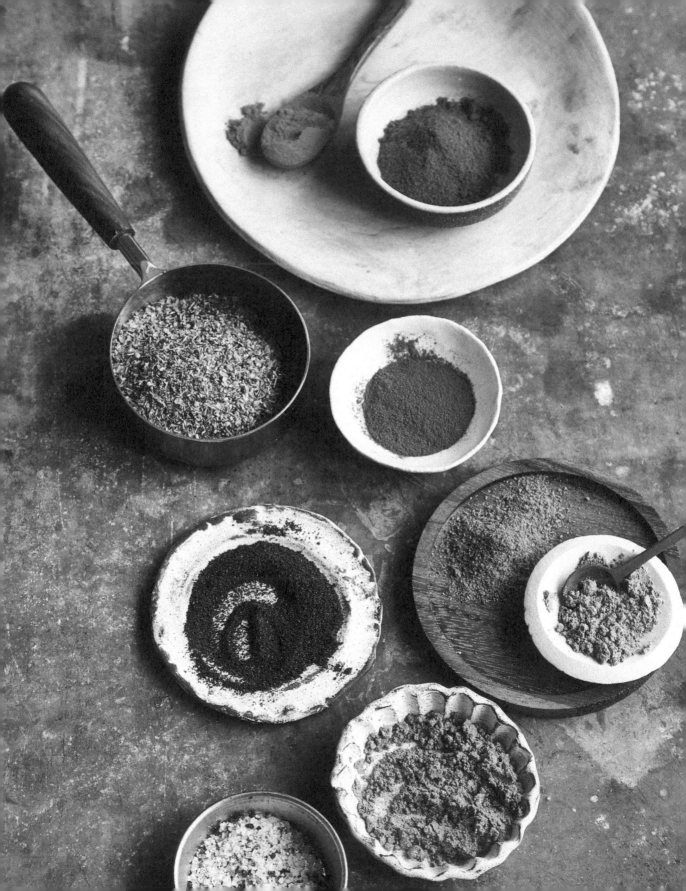

Measurement Conversions

	US STANDARD	US STANDARD (OUNCES)	METRIC (APPROXIMATE)
Volume Equivalents (Liquid)	2 tablespoons	1 fl. oz.	30 mL
	¼ cup	2 fl. oz.	60 mL
	½ cup	4 fl. oz.	120 mL
	1 cup	8 fl. oz.	240 mL
	1½ cups	12 fl. oz.	355 mL
	2 cups or 1 pint	16 fl. oz.	475 mL
	4 cups or 1 quart	32 fl. oz.	1 L
	1 gallon	128 fl. oz.	4 L
Volume Equivalents (Dry)	⅛ teaspoon	————	0.5 mL
	¼ teaspoon	————	1 mL
	½ teaspoon	————	2 mL
	¾ teaspoon	————	4 mL
	1 teaspoon	————	5 mL
	1 tablespoon	————	15 mL
	¼ cup	————	59 mL
	⅓ cup	————	79 mL
	½ cup	————	118 mL
	⅔ cup	————	156 mL
	¾ cup	————	177 mL
	1 cup	————	235 mL
	2 cups or 1 pint	————	475 mL
	3 cups	————	700 mL
	4 cups or 1 quart	————	1 L
	½ gallon	————	2 L
	1 gallon	————	4 L
Weight Equivalents	½ ounce	————	15 g
	1 ounce	————	30 g
	2 ounces	————	60 g
	4 ounces	————	115 g
	8 ounces	————	225 g
	12 ounces	————	340 g
	16 ounces or 1 pound	————	455 g

	FAHRENHEIT (F)	CELSIUS (C) (APPROXIMATE)
Oven Temperatures	250°F	120°F
	300°F	150°C
	325°F	180°C
	375°F	190°C
	400°F	200°C
	425°F	220°C
	450°F	230°C

Dirty Dozen™ and Clean Fifteen™

A nonprofit environmental watchdog organization called Environmental Working Group (EWG) looks at data supplied by the US Department of Agriculture (USDA) and the Food and Drug Administration (FDA) about pesticide residues. Each year it compiles a list of the best and worst pesticide loads found in commercial crops. You can use these lists to decide which fruits and vegetables to buy organic to minimize your exposure to pesticides and which produce is considered safe enough to buy conventionally. This does not mean they are pesticide-free, though, so wash these fruits and vegetables thoroughly. The list is updated annually, and you can find it online at EWG.org/FoodNews.

Dirty Dozen

1. strawberries
2. spinach
3. kale
4. nectarines
5. apples
6. grapes
7. peaches
8. cherries
9. pears
10. tomatoes
11. celery
12. potatoes

Additionally, nearly three-quarters of hot pepper samples contained pesticide residues.

Clean Fifteen

1. avocados
2. sweet corn*
3. pineapples
4. sweet peas (frozen)
5. onions
6. papayas*
7. eggplants
8. asparagus
9. kiwis
10. cabbages
11. cauliflower
12. cantaloupes
13. broccoli
14. mushrooms
15. honeydew melons

* A small amount of sweet corn, papaya, and summer squash sold in the United States is produced from genetically modified seeds. Buy organic varieties of these crops if you want to avoid genetically modified produce.

Resources

Clean Eating Kitchen is my website, which is devoted to gluten-free and dairy-free recipes and tips for women recovering from chronic disease. You can find my site at cleaneatingkitchen.com. Be sure to sign up for my weekly newsletter to get notified of the latest seasonal recipes and science-backed health tips.

The Institute for Functional Medicine has an online referral service to healthcare practitioners who are trained to look for the root cause of health problems, and who use nutrition and supplements to help treat health problems. I am a big fan of functional medicine, and it has been an essential part of my recovery from numerous health conditions. You can find the website at ifm.org.

Mercola.com is the website of Dr. Joseph Mercola, and it has numerous articles about natural health and wellness. I really admire Dr. Mercola and his team for their perspective on health, food, and wellness, which differs from the mainstream. If you are looking for information on more natural ways of living, I think you will like this site. Join Dr. Mercola's newsletter list to get free information delivered to your inbox.

Natural MD Radio is one of my favorite podcasts. The host, Dr. Aviva Romm, is an expert on women's health issues. Her website, avivaromm.com, is also excellent and includes information on how diet can affect hormones, weight issues, energy, and mental health.

US Wellness Meats is a great online source of grass-fed, organic, and naturally raised meats, poultry, and fish. Your order will arrive frozen on your doorstep. I have an extra freezer in my garage so I can order in bulk. Join their mailing list for recipes, discounts, interviews, and more. Visit the site at grasslandbeef.com.

Vitacost.com is my favorite online source for organic, natural, and healthy pantry items, supplements, cleaning supplies, and beauty products. I order from this site at least once a week. Sign up for their email list to get discounts. Visit Vitacost at vitacost.com.

Index

Acknowledgments

Thank you to my husband, Alan, for being so patient and supportive while I wrote two books in one year. You are an amazing person and life partner, and I'm so lucky to have you in my life. Thank you to my friends for keeping me motivated and sane throughout the process, including Janet, Scott, Francesca, Greta, Leah, Katey, and Emily. I am also hugely grateful to my blog audience, virtual friends, and social media followers, who share in my excitement and help me promote the book and my work. And, thank you to everyone at Callisto Media for helping me to write this book and making it a wonderful resource. Lastly, I acknowledge you, the reader, for your interest in leading a healthier life and all the steps that it takes to make that happen.

About the Author

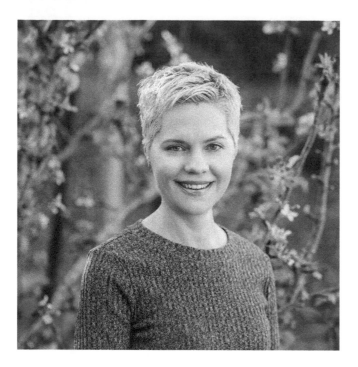

Carrie Forrest, MBA, MPH, is a clean eating specialist and creator of the website Clean Eating Kitchen, where she shares easy gluten-free and dairy-free recipes, and tips for women recovering from chronic health issues. Carrie has a professional background in nonprofit hospital fundraising and a master's degree in business and entrepreneurship from the University of Southern California.

Carrie became interested in nutrition to try to heal from a variety of health issues, including thyroid disease, digestive problems, chronic anxiety, migraines, PCOS, panic attacks, and multiple food sensitivities. She later earned a master's degree in public health nutrition from the University of Massachusetts at Amherst.

Carrie lives with her husband and two cats on California's beautiful central coast. When she's not testing, filming, and photographing recipes for her blog, she enjoys visiting farmers' markets, hiking, and learning to play the violin. Carrie can be reached on her blog, cleaneatingkitchen, on YouTube at Clean Eating Kitchen, or on Instagram @cleaneatingcarrie.

CPSIA information can be obtained
at www.ICGtesting.com
Printed in the USA
BVHW062102101219
565878BV00001BA/1/P